Dr Nikki Stamp FRACS is a cardiothoracic surgeon, one of only thirteen female heart surgeons in Australia. She has a strong desire to change the way we think about health by making it accessible and achievable. She is currently studying a PhD and has appeared as host of ABC TV's *Catalyst*, *Operation Live* and many other TV segments. Her writing has featured in *Washington Post*, *Mamamia*, *Sydney Morning Herald*, *Huffington Post* and *The Guardian*. *Scrubbed* is her third book.

Also by Dr Nikki Stamp
Can You Die of a Broken Heart?
Pretty Unhealthy

DR NIKKI STAMP

Scrubbed

A heart surgeon's
extraordinary memoir of
life, death and everything
in between

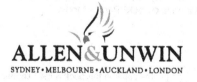

ALLEN&UNWIN
SYDNEY·MELBOURNE·AUCKLAND·LONDON

First published in 2022

Allen & Unwin
83 Alexander Street
Crows Nest NSW 2065
Australia
Phone: (61 2) 8425 0100
Email: info@allenandunwin.com
Web: www.allenandunwin.com

A catalogue record for this book is available from the National Library of Australia

ISBN 978 1 760879 41 9

Set in 12/18 pt Sabon LT STD by Midland Typesetters, Australia
Printed and bound in Australia by SOS Print + Media

10 9 8 7 6 5 4 3 2

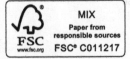

This book is dedicated to the true heroes in medicine—the patients and their loved ones. Thank you for your trust, your teaching and your inspiration that, despite the most challenging circumstances, give us all hope.

Contents

Disclaimer

Over the years, I have been privy to some of the most private moments of people's lives. Likewise, this book contains some things that I have seen and felt—my inner-most thoughts and fears, my experiences or those of my friends and colleagues—which I never thought I would share. All of the stories in this book are based on real events, but to protect everyone involved, names, details and times have been altered, and some stories are a blend of several experiences of my own and of other people's. Unless I have express permission from a person to include their name or story as it actually happened, I have taken artistic licence to keep secrets that need keeping.

The path of a surgeon

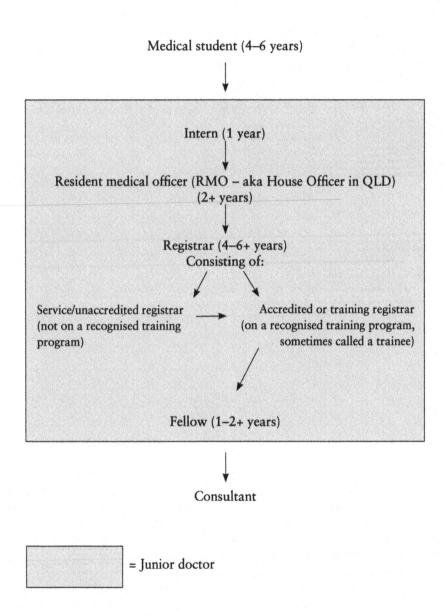

Medical student (4–6 years)

↓

Intern (1 year)

↓

Resident medical officer (RMO – aka House Officer in QLD)
(2+ years)

↓

Registrar (4–6+ years)
Consisting of:

Service/unaccredited registrar (not on a recognised training program) → Accredited or training registrar (on a recognised training program, sometimes called a trainee)

Fellow (1–2+ years)

↓

Consultant

▢ = Junior doctor

PREFACE

People often ask if working at a hospital is like TV.

Most people, thankfully, don't have much to do with someone like me. Let's be honest: nobody really wants to meet a heart surgeon, especially not as a patient. Most of what you think happens in a hospital might have come from watching George Clooney in *ER* or the interns of Seattle Grace Hospital using the on-call rooms for something other than sleeping in *Grey's Anatomy*. Maybe you recall seeing your local doctor, whiling away the time until your name was called, reading tabloid magazines that are at least five years out of date. In some doctor's waiting rooms, Prince William and Kate Middleton are still on a break.

I want you to disregard everything you think you know about life inside a hospital. There's no Dr House on a walking stick, hurling abuse at patients. No one is popping pills and getting his team to break into people's homes to diagnose something weird and wonderful. Nor is hospital life punctuated by a series of intense relationships between unbelievably good-looking colleagues, which are paused only occasionally to care for the sick and injured.

We're not the heroes that TV would have you believe, but that's not to say that life inside a hospital is any less interesting, at least some of the time. In reality, life inside a hospital and the experiences of people like me, I think, are far *more* interesting because they are real. Life in a hospital is everything from mundane to thrilling, with moments of even sheer terror or unbridled joy. There are definitely heroes in our midst but they lack the histrionics of the doctors on medical shows that so many people love.

For whatever reason, stories from medicine have always been popular except among doctors. Generally, doctors hate medical stories but we still consume those from our own. When I was in medical school, there was a book that all of the older doctors and professors told us to read because it was a 'real' look at what life was like inside medicine, away from the bright lights of Hollywood or the idealism that permeated medical school. (For more on the inner workings of an ICU, I highly suggest reading *Critical* by my friend and colleague Dr Matt Morgan.)

The House of God was written by Samuel Shem (the nom de plume of psychiatrist Stephen Bergman) and detailed the journey of a fresh-faced newly minted doctor as he navigated his early days in the profession. While he starts out naive and idealistic, his story twists and turns, diving into deep depression and reaching heady levels of ambition. Ultimately, in his fictionalised account of his first year as a doctor, he is ground down by the system. The politics, the loss of life and the dehumanisation of the protagonist ultimately culminate in Shem turning his back on hospital medicine to pursue a career in psychiatry where narcissism, callousness and a lack of care for one's own safety and wellbeing are notably (and happily) absent.

Among medical students and doctors, *The House of God* has a cult-like following. We recite lines from the book such as the 'Laws of the House of God', a set of thirteen salacious 'rules' born of cynicism for the system we work in. 'They can only hurt you more' or 'The only good admission is a dead admission' speak to the dark humour of the book but also are a result of a system that quite often erases any empathy for other people, particularly and most concerningly for your colleagues.

As we progress through our careers, *The House of God* sometimes goes from being a darkly satirical commentary on the pitfalls of the culture of medicine to being semi-autobiographical for many of us. I don't know very many doctors who hate medicine or wish to be removed from their patients and the altruism of our profession, but I know plenty who have been broken or damaged by the system. The politics of medicine, however, are what hurt us: the interpersonal nonsense, the inhumane hours and lack of sleep, the separation from our friends and family, the chronic underfunding of some areas of health care and the futility of fighting the bureaucracy.

During the COVID-19 pandemic, health care was thrust into the spotlight. All of a sudden, as the world grappled with a new normal, it became evident that doctors, nurses, orderlies, allied health staff—in fact, anyone who worked in health care—were facing an unfathomable task in defeating this pandemic. Globally, news outlets began running features on the brave front-line healthcare workers who were placing themselves at risk every day in COVID-19 wards. Thousands of healthcare workers around the world succumbed to the deadly infection.

Healthcare workers were suddenly the heroes of the hour. From the confines of lockdowns in countries everywhere, citizens stood on front doorsteps or balconies, cheering, clapping and banging pots and pans to thank heroic health-care workers. Social media was awash with praise for our bravery. Healthcare workers, including doctors, were showered with appreciation. The true stories of so-called 'healthcare heroes' finally eclipsed the manufactured and inaccurate medical shows that form the basis of so many people's beliefs about what happens behind our masks and under our drapes.

For me, COVID-19 happened at a very strange time in my life, a time when I was increasingly reflective about my career and where it was headed in the future. Watching the situation unfold, both from a scientific perspective and through the stories of our healthcare workers, gave me pause. It brought up many questions: about how we see doctors, about how little many people know of what we do outside a pandemic. While the sacrifices at this time were sometimes great and very public, many of us had already been giving all of ourselves even when we had very little left to give. COVID-19—the disease and the narrative—deepened my own reflections on my career, and my plans for the future.

* * *

What follows in the pages of this book has been, at times, deeply challenging to write. I've explored some of the darkness of our profession, through my own eyes and through the stories of other people—my friends, my colleagues and people I don't know personally but whose experiences touched me somehow. And I've also remembered some of the most brilliant times of my career, celebrated wins with my patients or my colleagues and remembered the heady adoration I have for the human body, much like I did when I was a child.

When I started writing this book, I actually didn't know how it was going to end. I didn't know if the final chapter would see me walking away from the career I had once cared about so much or whether I would be reinvigorated and open to new opportunities. The stories in these pages are big, with big emotions, and the ending is no different.

I wonder what the little girl who obsessed over the pages of books about the human body would think of everything that has happened since. Despite the roller-coaster ride that this has been to date, despite the hard times, I really hope that if she knew where her love of medicine would take her, she would do it anyway.

The reason I didn't know how this book would end is that while I was writing it, I couldn't say with confidence that I would want her to.

INTRODUCTION
My heart's desire

I remember when I first wanted to become a doctor. I was around seven or eight years old. My school library had a small collection of books on the human body, grouped into systems: *The Heart, The Eye and Vision, The Skeletal System.* I knew them all, every single one, off by heart. I knew how light passes through the cornea, the thin layer at the front of the eye, before passing through the lens, which both focuses and inverts the image, which then lands on your retina at the back of the eye. From there, the rods and cones translate that light signal into little electrical impulses to your brain so that you can see.

I knew that cells lumped together make tissues, and when we put tissues together they in turn make an organ. Livers, hearts and lungs can all be broken down in this very predictable way to the smallest of building blocks. Specialised muscle cells, called myocytes, have microscopic filaments inside them that act like a pulley system to shorten the cells and in turn the whole muscle, moving the limbs. The cells that line the gut have little finger-like projections that jut out into the bowel, allowing those cells to mop up everything it can to keep us nourished. The thigh bone is actually called the femur and your forearm has two bones that rotate around one another as your wrist turns back and forth. And the heart was created before we were born, out of a single tube that twisted and danced upon itself to give us four chambers of a fully formed heart.

I consumed these books with a burning fascination and eventually I decided to branch out and read the St John's First Aid manual, where I learnt how to treat someone who was choking—by a forceful blow (or several), delivered right between the shoulder blades. I knew that if someone had a hole in their chest (called an open pneumothorax) that was sucking in air, the way to fix that was to take a piece of plastic and tape it over the wound, leaving one edge open. This would act as a one-way valve to let air escape while stopping more getting in, preventing the lung from collapsing further and the patient dying. I knew how many breaths to chest compressions were needed to give cardiopulmonary resuscitation (CPR) to someone.

Around that time, I remember one night there was a commotion on the street and my mum went to the house across the road, thinking that our neighbour was deathly ill. This was my chance to put into practice everything

I had learnt. I was ready to step up and save a life with my extensive medical knowledge. It was a heady mix of excitement and calm in with a—perhaps misplaced—sense of purpose. (Even now, this exact feeling pops up again from time to time.)

Did I mention I was eight years old?

I suppose I can concede now that I was probably not as ready as I thought I was. As it turned out, I never got the chance to apply my skills and knowledge as a child prodigy. In fact, it wasn't until medical school, much later, that I would experience that feeling again, when you know you're on the thin line that exists between life and death or pain and comfort. Now, I can reflect on that unwavering obsession and see it as endearing; without fail it brings a smile to my face to know that I have always loved something that much.

I don't know where this obsession came from. There were no doctors or nurses in my family. My dad was an engineer; my mum had been a flight attendant, in the days when the crew aspired to look like Farah Fawcett. Nonetheless, there was something magnetic about the human body to me and I was beyond excited to learn how it worked and desperate to fix it when it failed.

I used to see a man by the name of Dr Victor Chang on TV. He was a cardiac surgeon in Sydney who most notably transplanted one of Australia's youngest-ever heart transplant recipients. He was our nation's hero, working on a durable mechanical heart to replace the amazing yet incredibly flawed process of a heart transplant. I may have known about retinas and bones, or where the kidneys were located, but if I had one true love, even at that time, it was the human heart.

Around this time, my grandfather started to get unwell. He was a gruff man, probably a function of growing up in London, surviving the blitz and serving in the Royal British Navy. He used to stomp around his house and lose his temper at my brother and me when we made too much noise, which was often when I was around. But over the course of a few weeks, he started to tire easily and became noticeably kinder, an alert to the fact that something was wrong. It was not long after this that he was diagnosed with an aggressive form of cancer called mesothelioma. It's a cancer of the lining of the chest cavity, called the pleura, and it is caused by exposure to asbestos. He deteriorated rapidly over the course of months, needing regular pleural taps, where a small tube is placed into the chest under local anaesthetic to drain the fluid that was squashing his lungs, stealing his breath.

I detailed his medical care in my school journal: how he needed a few litres of bloody fluid drained away every couple of weeks; how he was on a trial medication that my dad injected into his abdomen a few nights a week, trying to stop the cancer that enveloped his lungs from suffocating him from the inside. It was a last desperate attempt to save, or at least prolong, his life—or, at the very least, learn something of how this treatment would help others. My school journal became like medical notes in a hospital, the ones kept on each and every patient.

My grandfather died only a few months after his diagnosis. I look back on that now and wonder if his intense contact with the medical profession at that time fanned the flames of my desire for a medical career. Aside from the care he received at home, I never really saw his doctors or ventured into the hospital with him. But the idea of facing this invisible enemy, learning about it and then battling it, hopefully defeating it like a dragon in a fairytale, clearly grabbed hold of me. And at eight years old, I made the daring assertion that when I grew up, I was going to be a heart surgeon and finish the work of Dr Victor Chang. No ballerina or princess aspirations here: heart surgery was the only way forward for me.

As I got older, my fascination with learning in general waned. I don't know if that was because I swapped paying attention in class and completing homework for the feeble rebellion of ignoring lessons and clamouring for the attention and approval of my more popular classmates, but all of a sudden, excelling in academia was not a priority. And like most teenagers, I began a years-long flip-flop of career options, from lawyer to journalist to actor to accountant. My report cards all began to say the exact same thing: 'Nikki talks too much and does not apply herself,' a marker of the frustration I caused my parents and my teachers who knew I was capable of much more. My Year 10 maths teacher went one step further and told my parents that because of my lack of mathematical aptitude, I'd never be anything important like a doctor or a lawyer. (She was half right; I'm not a lawyer. Yet.)

At that time, I didn't see that I was not using my potential; what I saw was that I was not smart enough. I was blinded by my underperformance, which really only came from a lack of application rather than a lack of ability. And so, I chose a career that I was intensely passionate about, in musical theatre. However, by the time Year 12 came around, my dad had grown increasingly uncomfortable with my dreams of Broadway and the West End and insisted that I get a 'real degree' first, a sensible back-up career in case my dreams of treading the boards failed to actualise. And I chose accounting, the most sensible of all the sensible careers.

As my high school days drew to a close, I was increasingly uncomfortable with this choice. Not because I desperately wanted to forgo my back-up plan for a shot at the bright lights of stage and screen but because I knew I did not want to be an accountant, not even as a back-up plan. So, my dad and I spent hours poring over the offerings of every university, trying to find something I'd prefer. Each time I flicked past the pages on medicine, something grabbed me. I was completely unaware of why that was, having long since forgotten my utter obsession with the human body.

As I got increasingly frustrated, because I didn't think I would have the marks necessary for one option or I hadn't done the necessary prerequisite subjects for another, my dad took away all the brochures and asked me, if I could do anything in the world, no matter the marks or subjects, what would I do. And I surprised myself when, without hesitation, I announced that I would want to be a doctor. This was immediately followed by a sense of devastation. I had under-performed, just as my teachers had warned I would. I had missed the medical school entrance exams; I had dropped chemistry.

My stubborn streak took over here as I set about finding a way to study medicine and discovered that I could study science and then apply a year later to medical school. And the number of people, just like my maths teacher, who told me I would never do it, that I wasn't smart enough, that the odds were not in my favour, grew all the time. As it turned out, they were very wrong. I was smart enough; in fact, after just one year of studying chemistry and science and all of the things I thought I wasn't good enough to do, I got into medical school.

It turned out, in hindsight, that my eight-year-old self knew what my true love was all along.

PART I

Scrubbing in

1

INTERN

Shit and assholes

CASE 1

The elevator doors slide open and behind them, a young woman is kneeling on a gurney desperately pushing life into the chest of a man. She yells out pointed commands as she straddles him while the trolley thunders out of the elevator down a stark white hospital corridor.

'Push epi!'

'Come on! We're losing him!'

'Don't die on me, not today!'

A nurse pulls the paddles from the defibrillator. She shouts 'Charging!', rubbing the paddles together while the machine screams as it winds up to 240 joules.

'Clear!' she shouts once more as the young doctor throws her hands up in the air and the nurse pushes the paddles onto the seemingly dead man's chest, discharging the full force of electricity that will perform a kind of hard reset on his heart. His body bucks on the bed as the electricity courses through him. And it works. The man coughs and splutters and the doctor dismounts from the gurney, looking satisfied.

'Another life saved, doc,' says the stalwart and knowing orderly. She turns to him with a wry grin and says, 'Another? It's my first day.' Her bouncy blonde locks swirl around her as she struts down the corridor on her very first day as a shiny new intern as the opening credits roll over a catchy indie tune.

CRITICAL REFLECTION QUESTION
What do you observe about the life of an intern in this case study?

This is how interns begin their medical careers, or so TV would have you believe. This generic introduction to the earnest and talented new doctor is common fodder for virtually all medical shows. Our new superheroes may as well put their undies on the outside as they start their first day in the hospital where they'll fight for patients, they'll fight the system and they'll win your heart.

I feel like it goes without saying that medical shows stretch the truth more than a little. For me, my medical career started with a whimper, not a bang. There was no cardiac arrest, no cool theme song, no Patrick Dempsey or Zach Braff. On my very first day as a doctor on the orthopaedic ward, it didn't take long for me to come up against the reality that the world of medicine is decidedly unglamorous.

CASE 2

'Hi Nikki, I'm Marie; I'm the nurse looking after Bed 72. Could you chart some aperients, please?' Marie had found me in the doctors' office on the ward, where I was wrangling with a computer to check the blood results for patients. The computers were still running an outdated version of Windows and were painfully slow. In the years that followed, the IT never got any better.

'Absolutely,' I responded with all the confidence of a fictional TV doctor, 'I'll bring the chart back to you in a moment.'

When Marie had left the doctors' office and was well out of earshot, I asked my fellow interns what the hell aperients were. These were the days before everyone had smart phones, on which I could have discreetly looked up what Marie was after. (Yes, I've been a doctor for that long.) I was informed that they were medications to help you defecate (not in such delicate terms). Obviously, I knew what laxatives were and how to prescribe them; I had just never heard of the term aperients before. And that was how my medical career began: a shitty start. Literally.

CRITICAL REFLECTION QUESTION
What do you observe about the life of an intern in this
case study? How does it compare to the first case?

I was studious at medical school, which is a polite way of
saying that I hung around like a bad smell. I was there late
at night, on weekends, on holidays, asking questions and
offering help, although at that stage I don't know whether I
was a help or a hindrance on account of my inexperience.
I was the student who was always knee-deep in patients'
notes and almost always knew the answer to the question
that the professor asked. If you are a fan of the sitcom *Scrubs*,
I was Elliot. I knew how to hand-tie sutures (a vital skill for
a budding surgeon) and even then, the operating theatre was
my Disneyland: the happiest place on Earth. I *loved* medical
school, although I don't think 'love' actually captures just how
much I was completely and utterly captivated by learning the
art and science of medicine.

I say this not to brag that I was some hot-shot med student
who was destined for greatness. In fact, thinking back to my
medical school friends, we were all studious, diligent and
committed to be the best that we could possibly be. I wasn't
as special as it sounds. I point this out to say that I was not
at all underprepared to be an actual doctor. I was more than
ready and entirely capable on the first day I stepped onto
that orthopaedic ward as an intern.

For many people, the grades and stages of doctors make about as much sense as whatever jargon the doctor uses to explain what the hell is going on with your body. It goes a little something like this. An intern is a doctor the first year out of medical school and it's a year of closely supervised practice, although you're a licensed doctor. That year, you rotate every couple of months or so, giving you a broad experience in internal medicine, surgery and emergency medicine. After that, you are a resident medical officer (RMO) and it is at this time that we start to stream towards our final destination. The surgically inclined doctors start to make their rounds on rotations of all the various surgical specialties, the internal medicine fans do the same and so on. Normally, we spend a couple of years or more at this 'rank'.

Once you've made the biggest decision of your life— what to specialise in—you become a registrar, which is known as a resident in North America. Yes, I know: some may disagree with me here as to whether this is the biggest decision of your life. Maybe you think it's choosing a spouse or having children and that's fine. But this is a massive deal.

It's when you are a registrar that things start to get serious, where your days (and nights) are spent at the hospital, or in community practice if you're going to be a general practitioner, working as a kind of apprentice. And once you've worked a ten- to twelve-hour day (or longer), you get to go home, mumble at your family/spouse/housemate/dog and then settle in for the night with your mobile phone to be on call or dive into a nice thick textbook and pile of scientific journal articles to learn every inch of your chosen specialty. Getting to this point is tough, with selection for specialty training getting more and more fierce by the year. Some registrars aren't even actually formally training in their specialty.

Like RMOs, registrars can rotate through every few months, gaining extra experience and marking time until they can get accepted to a training program. These registrars are called service or unaccredited registrars; those lucky enough to be accepted into a training program are called trainees or accredited registrars. Some doctors spend several years as unaccredited registrars before getting accepted as an official trainee and some never get the chance to advance.

At the end of your training time, which could be up to ten years (or more) after you leave medical school no matter what you specialise in, you are faced with some very scary, very challenging and very expensive (to the tune of $8000) exams called fellowship exams. They are designed to prove that you are safe and competent as an independent specialist. Once you pass this final hurdle, you are a consultant (an 'attending' in North America) or a specialist in your chosen field. We sometimes call this 'getting your letters' because you are generally then awarded a fellowship of a college, so you get to add some more letters to the alphabet soup that comes after your name; my letters are FRACS or Fellow of the Royal Australasian College of Surgeons.

It's the antipodean equivalent of being 'board certified' and costs more money yet again, to the tune of several thousand dollars just to register your name. Becoming a specialist is not a cheap or easy exercise.

But I have gotten way ahead of myself here, because before you can get your letters, you need to prescribe some laxatives (aka aperients) for Marie's patient in Bed 72 who hasn't had the pleasure of a good bowel motion for a couple of days. (Hospital staff often refer to people by bed numbers or 'the woman with the femur fracture', which I have to say, I really hate. It's so impersonal and was one of the things I promised myself I would try desperately hard not to do, and most of the time I keep that promise.)

This is the reality of intern life. Before the heady success of letters and the immense stress of exams comes the banality of rewriting medication charts, carefully transcribing the professor's ward-round instructions and being a slave to your pager. Hospitals are one of the last remaining bastions of technology that belong in the 1980s—for some reason we are still enslaved to pagers and fax machines despite mobile phones and email being far superior technology. (Incidentally, pagers are quite possibly the most infuriating sound in the universe. I won't lie: I fantasised about putting mine under the back wheel of my car or dropping it in the toilet. But I didn't because rumour was that the hospital would charge you to replace it.)

My complaints about pagers and deciphering colleagues' handwriting to diligently copy a patient's medications to a new chart when the old one runs out of space is not to trivialise the role of the intern. It's to contrast it with the romanticised expectations of heroics that swim around the heads of new recruits or take centre stage in medical dramas. The reality of life inside a hospital, especially as you find your feet in those early days, is one of paperwork and phone calls. Without them, the hospital and the patient's care would grind to a screeching halt.

A good intern is like a point guard on a basketball team, or a wicketkeeper. They can be the glue that holds every-thing together, enabling the rest of their team to do their jobs efficiently, untroubled by the minutiae of hospital life that seems trivial but is actually as important as anything else. A good intern is the patient's ally since they are often on the ward more than the rest of the doctors on the team, who beaver away in theatre or see people in clinics. Interns are in the trenches, so to speak, with the nurses who are also there at the bedside much more than a consultant like me. A good intern will also help a consultant like me who cannot for the life of her work out which one of the thousands of computer programs I need to use to order a chest X-ray. That's when a good intern will gently push my wheelie chair away from the computer and take over because she can't stand to watch my IT ineptitude any longer.

I could probably divide my cohort of interns into two groups: either confident and ready to go or 'Holy shit, they made me a doctor?' Whichever way you leant, most of us, regardless of underlying ethos, were a bit petrified of emergency medicine. After all, this was where you were most likely to be in the thick of something terrifying or exciting, depending on your outlook on life. I loved emergency medicine, so much so that it crossed my mind to leave my surgical dreams behind to be a wannabe cast member of *ER*.

Back when I was an intern, the ED—the Emergency Department—was where you cut your teeth as a doctor. The department was invariably busy, with sick patients, weird and wonderful presentations and an opportunity for our interventions to legitimately save a life. When things really get dramatic, the ED is about as close to TV medicine as you get in a hospital. The team in ED—whether it be doctors, nurses, support staff—thrives off the chaos and unpredictability of emergency medicine, never knowing what will come through the door next. And they were all really, really great at it.

ED was the place where you got to actually *do* a whole bunch of cool things as an intern, not just paperwork. It's where I got to put my burgeoning surgical skills into practice on a Saturday and Sunday morning when the people who had been out drinking the night before had sobered up enough to have their wounds stitched. I loved hiding out in the little procedure room suturing heads, arms, even ears— battle scars from a night that had been either really good or really bad.

I used to wait for the sound of the 'bat phone'—a red phone with a flashing light that was the direct line from

ambulances, on which they'd give us a forewarning of a critically unwell patient coming our way. This was the warning
used for massive strokes, cardiac arrests or major trauma.
I always rushed to be the intern for those patients; in my
youthful exuberance I sometimes forgot that my exciting
interesting thing was actually the worst day of their life.
Being amid the suffering that a bat phone call could bring
knocked that out of me quick smart.

One of my consultants realised that I had an affinity
for the bat phone and she chastised me for cherry-picking
the 'full-on cases', leaving the less adrenaline-inducing
ones. I denied it, but she was absolutely right. But I absolutely loved those cases; in the thick of those critical cases
was where I felt most like a doctor. Years later, in answer
to overcrowding, the 'four-hour rule' was introduced,
whereby patients in ED needed to be admitted or discharged
within the magic timeframe. I lamented that rule because
I knew, had that been in place when I was an intern, the
focus may have shifted from teaching to reaching a target.
While overcrowding in EDs is a genuine patient safety
issue, the four-hour rule has its drawbacks as well as its
good points.

ED was also the only place I saw a fellow intern try to
emulate TV medicine, when a patient in full cardiac arrest
was wheeled from the ambulance entrance to the resuscitation bays of the department with an intern atop giving
CPR. The consultant emergency physician that day, a battle-
hardened former military doctor, yelled, 'Who the fuck is

that and what the fuck is he doing?' then proceeded to pull the guy off the patient. (I assume my fellow intern got a very stern talking to afterwards.) This particular consultant was always straight to the point, the pressing nature of emergency medicine meaning they had no time for stuffing around or pretending like you were on *Grey's Anatomy*.

Our inner-city hospital was exactly where an ED should be, in the heart of where people needed us. It served some of the most disadvantaged areas, people who had nowhere to live and those who struggled with addiction, while also close to the night-life districts where, almost inevitably, come Saturday night fights would break out and injuries would ensue. The hospital also backed onto a train line, the same one I'd catch to and from work when I could.

ED was where I got my first needlestick injury as a doctor. Late on a Friday night, the police had brought in a young man whom they thought was under the influence of some kind of substance. But they weren't sure whether his combativeness and slurred speech might be due to some illness, so he was brought to us to make sure he didn't have a medical problem. We didn't know what he had done to become so friendly with the police; it was not really ours to know.

I was instructed to take bloods from the young man, who had gone from being allegedly combative with the police to lying back in the hospital gurney, blankly staring at the ceiling. As I approached him, he didn't move his gaze at all. I wondered what he had taken or perhaps what was so interesting on the ceiling. I entered the tiny cubicle and explained to him that I needed to take some blood from him to make sure he wasn't sick and asked him if it was okay. He briefly looked at me and nodded his agreement, before turning back to the ceiling.

As I got close and put the tourniquet around his right arm, I could smell the alcohol on his breath, not unusual for a weekend night. 'Sharp scratch!' I warned him as I plunged the needle into the vein inside the elbow on his right arm and withdrew the blood. He barely moved, even when the needle pierced his skin. But as I went to loosen the tourniquet, he moved; he moved quite a lot. He took the syringe, needle still attached, out of his arm and stuck it into the fleshy part of my hand, just below my left thumb. It took me a second to register what had happened but as I realised I'd just had a high-risk needlestick injury, I yelled out for help. The police and security guards descended on the cubicle and the once-quiet man thrashed about as they struggled to contain his violent kicks. I just watched, aghast, until one of the nurses whisked me away. For my troubles, I wound up with six weeks of anti-retroviral treatment in case he had HIV that he had passed along to me. For the remainder of the shift, although he had been sedated for his and our safety, I gave the cubicle a wide berth and brushed off the constant pitying querying from the department staff. Yes, I was fine. No, I didn't need to go home. No, I definitely did not need to talk to anyone.

ED felt like real medicine. You made diagnoses of everything from major traumas to pneumonia to broken bones of every variety. It was fast and dirty medicine where you had to quickly work out what was going on and start some treatment asap. And the treatment would most often work in front of your eyes: someone's pain would disappear or their oxygen levels would normalise or even their bleeding would subside.

But although I loved the excitement and busyness of life in the ED, it was never for me, not really. Not least of all because my heart already belonged to surgery but also because I hated not knowing what happened to people. After the ED, patients would then make their way to their final destinations. Lung problems went to the respiratory ward, heart attacks to the coronary care unit. Some people were whisked away to operating theatres for lifesaving surgery. Some people went straight home. It always seemed to be a case of out of sight, out of mind. Not because people didn't care, but because, once that person had left, there were dozens more who needed our attention. That not knowing, or not being involved beyond those few hours or even minutes, drove me crazy. I always wanted to know what happened.

EDs sometimes have patients called 'frequent flyers'—people who present repeatedly, often with the same problem. They know the staff by name and the staff know almost everything about them in turn. Most of these people were not necessarily perpetually ill. Some were homeless and lived in the hostels or on the streets surrounding my inner-city hospital. Coming to ED was a place to get a cup of tea, some sandwiches and a bed for the night. (It took me a while to realise that that was why they were coming to hospital and it was when I first started to realise the world could be desperately unfair to some people.)

I remember one patient distinctly. His name was Mr Happy. That was his actual legal name; he'd changed it some years before and there were half a dozen stories as to why he had. He'd been high; he'd been drunk; he'd been a stage performer in a circus. Mr Happy came to ED at least once or twice a week, usually saying he had chest pain. Chest pain is a good symptom to say because you'll never be turned away in case we miss you having a heart attack. We had a management plan for Mr Happy; he would be checked by the doctors and nurses to ensure he wasn't having a heart attack, he'd get some painkillers, his cup of tea and sandwiches and a bed for the night. The next morning, the social worker would try to make sure he was safe and then he would be discharged. We'd always see him again soon.

I used to see Mr Happy on a bench a few hundred metres down the road from the hospital when I was walking to the train station or into town for food. He was often asleep; his frequent companion was a bottle of something, half hidden in a paper bag. I would be saddened and relieved, usually in equal measure, to see him there. Saddened because what kind of life do we let people lead that this is their refuge, a bench on a city street? Relieved because he was okay and would inevitably be back at one of my next shifts.

I moved on from ED to another department of the hospital, as is standard for interns, but I still continued the same walk. For a few weeks, I'd noticed Mr Happy's bench was occupied by strangers: no bottle, no Mr Happy. The next time I was in ED, I asked one of the senior nurses what had happened to him.

'He finally died,' she said, completely straight-faced.

I don't know what I felt: perhaps sadness at a life lived on a park bench, mitigated only by occasional respite at a bustling hospital ED (with, let's be honest, the worst sandwiches you were ever likely to be subjected to). I was also angry that that was someone's life. What the hell did that say about us as a society? What did it say about him?

But the nurse had been so detached. Not that she didn't care: she had the most beautiful bedside manner with her patients and her colleagues alike. I never told her, but she was my favourite nurse and remained so even years after I left the ED. Was a lifetime in a hospital that jading that someone's passing was only to be remarked upon without emotion? Is that the only way to survive the chaos—detachment? Would that be me one day?

About halfway into my intern year, I finally made it to my general surgical rotation. By this stage, I thought I was doing pretty well. I didn't need to ask anyone what aperients were, for example. I was unbelievably excited to be in surgery again. And I was lucky enough to be on the upper gastrointestinal (GI) team—the best general surgery team in the hospital (this is an entirely subjective assessment but I loved the surgeries they did so I stand by my assessment). GI had the slickest surgeons but also the most demanding ones. One of the consultants used to mandate that 'all the boys must wear ties'. 'Boys' was used to refer to all the junior doctors, male or female, a habit not unique to this surgeon. (A tie never really went with my outfit.) We were expected to fall in line and work hard, for free. There was a letter from the head of the department telling interns and residents not to claim any overtime—basically, work for free because you love it and claiming overtime would be unwise, unless you wanted a bad reference and a reputation as a troublemaker. This letter and this attitude about overtime were not unique to surgery; it was a profession-wide ethos.

I used to come into work at least an hour or two before my scheduled start time, to get my paperwork done for the day to free me up to sneak off to the operating theatre so I could learn how to suture, how to do a laparotomy (if I was very lucky) or even be the first assistant to the registrars or the consultant during a big surgery. The first assistant felt like a second-in-command to me then. They're there to help the operating surgeon do the surgery and, sometimes, that meant putting in actual sutures or using the instruments like I actually knew what to do with them.

My early starts also allowed me to prepare for ward rounds with a consultant widely known for his high expectations. (The same guy who mandated ties.) I would try to memorise every patient's blood test results: their haemoglobin, their white cell count. I'd check their X-rays or CT scans and make a note of what had been found. The number that he was always obsessed with though, and the number I always made a point of remembering above all else, was the potassium. Potassium is one of the electrolytes in the body, and in patients who have had surgery or who have an illness the potassium can be all over the place. This is very problematic; a potassium level that is too high or too low can cause deadly heart problems.

On one particular day, the boss turned up to the ward round carrying his breakfast, as he always did, a habit of a lifetime of having to eat on the run. So many of our patients were fasting in preparation for surgery or to let their bowel heal after an operation, and it always struck me as strange that he would stand outside their room eating, the very thing I was pretty sure many of them would have murdered for. That day I was distracted by the breakfast sandwich, so I initially didn't hear him grilling me.

'Nikki, why have you prescribed paracetamol IV?' In those days, IV—or intravenous—paracetamol was a relatively new drug and being able to give it that way rather than by a tablet was like a shiny new toy, especially for our poor unfed patients. And that was the reason that I offered up. 'Because they're fasting, Mr X,' I said. (In some states of Australia and in the UK, surgeons are called 'Mr' as a throwback to the days when surgeons were barbers or butchers and not doctors. I hate the term—it's gendered and confusing.)

'Do you know how much this costs?' he asked me. I shook my head, as he rattled the glass vial hanging from a drip stand by the patient's bed. 'Today, you're going to go down to pharmacy and find out how much IV paracetamol costs in comparison to PR paracetamol. Because the only excuse for not giving PR paracetamol is that the patient doesn't have an asshole.'

You're the only asshole right here, I thought to myself. Because advocating for having the patients go through a suppository in their rectum (PR means 'per rectum') seemed kind of mean. I actually didn't really think he was an asshole, not at all. He demanded excellence and although he had just chewed me out, me calling him that, even in my head, was not a reflection of who he actually was.

Reeling from the PR paracetamol meant that when we got around to the next patient, I was off my game, seething from the slapping I had just received. Mr X may have sensed it and started to quiz me about this man's blood test results. He had undergone a huge operation called a Whipple's procedure a few days prior, meaning his pancreas, spleen and part of his duodenum (the first portion of the gut after the stomach) had been removed. These patients can be very sick and monitoring their bloods means we can trouble-shoot before things get too bad. Haemoglobin 96. White cell count 12. Creatinine 86. Potassium . . . potassium. Shit, I had forgotten it.

Mr X quizzed the registrar, who had not looked at the bloods because as the intern, it was my job to be balls deep in blood test results. He had no idea either and so, there again, we both got a bollocking. At least this time the misery was shared around.

Although I was perturbed, I was not really offended. Mr X was one of the surgeons in my first few years of being a doctor who pushed me and I liked the pressure. It drives me, if only so that I can never again be asked the price difference between IV and PR paracetamol without knowing the answer. And so that I am fully aware of the gravity of what we do. The quizzing was possibly a little for entertainment, to exert some power and test me for fun. But predominantly it was so I didn't for a second forget the seriousness of what we did there, because that's how we were all taught; nobody knew any better. Mr X was one of the surgeons whose early pushing made me what I am today. And now he's my colleague, I know he's happy when I've turned up to share the operating table with him when his cases have needed a cardiac surgeon.

While some of my peers hated that kind of pressure, I relished it. It was an opportunity for me to rise to the occasion. I set high standards for myself, so when someone raised them even higher I didn't see it as an inconvenience, I saw it as a challenge, a gauntlet thrown. Usually the consultants that everyone else would openly call assholes were the ones that I loved. The consultants that my friends detested for their unrelenting standards I just wanted to please. I wanted to be pushed; I wanted to be challenged because I wanted to be the best. So Mr X and anyone else like him may have irritated me momentarily from time to time, but in reality, I loved the pressure. I thrived on it and I respected the hell out of them. I didn't realise at the time that maybe

I had just drunk my first cup of Kool-Aid, that this wasn't the way a medical workplace needed to be. Or maybe I just told myself that this was okay in order to survive.

Either way, I couldn't wait to be just like them.

2

RESIDENT MEDICAL OFFICER

The way of the heart

My intern year was a stand-out year in so many respects. Finally graduating, finally working as a doctor, making new friends and learning so much. Being an intern is the first year of your apprenticeship, learning a little about a lot and cementing all the skills. I felt like a sponge that year, lapping up every bit of knowledge that I could. But, just as I had been as a child, I was a precocious intern. I just wanted to grow up to be a big girl surgeon.

In Australia, after your successful intern year, doctors start to stream towards their chosen field as resident medical officers, known as RMOs or residents. (Except in Queensland, where you're called a house officer, a throwback to our colonial history. Why the state insists on using this nomenclature is beyond me; the medical hierarchy is confusing enough as it is for patients.) Your time as an RMO usually lasts two or three years, depending on the person and the place. The internal medicine kids start delving into all the physician specialties like cardiology, rheumatology or respiratory medicine. The doctors who love critical care will head towards the intensive care unit, to be serenaded by endless numbers of machines that go ping, supporting lives that hang in the balance. The future paediatricians pack up their bubbles and toy puppets and head to a kids' hospital and the future obstetricians move to the labour ward, ready to catch a baby or two.

The surgeons are, of course, no different. We wave good-bye to our colleagues and teachers in these other specialties, swapping what are often called our clinical clothes—the smart business casual that makes us look like 'real professional doctors' for the industrially laundered, perpetually ill fitting and often itchy surgical scrubs. Hospital scrubs are also not made for women so they fit us in an even less flattering way, if that's possible. We run screaming from the wards to the safe spaces of the operating theatres, where we jostle and position ourselves to scrub into surgeries to learn the basics (and beyond) of surgery.

While I loved being an intern, I didn't love being a resident. I was too hungry for the next rung up the career ladder. As an RMO, you were still a bottom feeder of sorts, relegated to the unglamorous jobs of medicine like paperwork, collecting X-ray films (when I was an RMO, a good number of X-rays were still printed out on the black and grey plastic that younger readers have probably only seen in movies, whereas now they are almost entirely digital) for department meetings and very much lowest in the pecking order. I was ambitious and all I wanted was to keep marching my way towards my life as a consultant surgeon. But, as badly as I wanted the end results, I had to do my time just like everyone else.

RMOs rotate through different specialties, depending on what your career path is. My resident year was my first year of basic surgical training so I spent the whole year dipping in and out of various surgical specialties and critical care, like intensive care, all geared towards making me the most well-rounded surgeon I could be. It was the year I learnt the most surgical procedures. I learnt how to reduce a fracture and drill broken bones in orthopaedics and how to perform a cystos-copy (placing a camera up the urethra—the hole you pee out of—to look inside a bladder) and many other procedures.

Despite everything that I was gaining, I was consumed by ambition as I continued my march towards being an actual, real-life surgeon. My friends took a year off to go and work in the UK as a kind of working holiday but I was worried that, by doing so, I'd set myself back a year in my quest for surgical greatness. So while they experienced life elsewhere, I stayed put with my head down, soldiering on towards my end goal.

When I was an RMO, I had my heart set on ortho-paedic surgery—surgery of the bones and joints, thanks in large part due to my mum's experience. When she was just forty years old, she was diagnosed with a particularly aggressive form of arthritis. It was diagnosed late as doctor after doctor told her that her inability to walk was 'all in her head' or just because she was a bored housewife. In the years since, she's had dozens of joint replacements or other surgeries and some days even the most basic tasks are excruciating. In hindsight, my mum was a big influence on my career— I wanted to fix her and people like her and I definitely wanted to ensure that patients wouldn't be dismissed like she had been.

With everyone clamouring for their favourite rotation, the task of allocating hundreds of doctors to their dream rotation was no easy task, and so we often had to negotiate with the matriarch of medical administration, a lady by the name of Joyce. She was so well known that even doctors from overseas knew you had to be nice to Joyce in order to get the jobs you wanted. She was so sharp and knew everyone, including what your career aspirations were. But she never gave you what you wanted just because you asked, or even begged her for it. You had to help her out as well, filling some of the less popular positions in exchange for the ones you'd give your right arm for. My negotiation involved getting my eleven weeks in my beloved orthopaedic surgery in exchange for what I assumed was going to be a painful and unfulfilling term in cardiothoracic surgery. (I had clearly forgotten my childhood aspirations and obsessions.)

When I landed in cardiothoracic surgery, I loudly announced to anyone in earshot that I was simply passing through, doing my duty so that I could get back to my dream job—orthopaedics. Little by little, though, cardiac surgery began to seduce me. Cardiac surgery is somewhat unusual among surgical specialties in that it combines the technical grace of operating with the in-depth knowledge you would expect of a physician. A physician is a doctor who practices internal medicine—they tend to use medications to treat disease, such as an oncologist giving chemotherapy. Physicians are reputed to have almost encyclopaedic knowledge of their area of expertise. A surgeon performs actual surgeries, operations on your insides, and is often an expert in anatomy—where everything can be found in your body, although this is a slight oversimplification on both sides. (The physician counterpart of a cardiothoracic surgeon is a cardiologist, who does tests to diagnose heart conditions and uses medications, although some will perform less invasive procedures like heart stents.)

Cardiothoracic surgeons don't just know where everything is; we can describe in great detail the intricacies of how the heart actually works. I once heard cardiac surgeons called 'physicians who operate', a nod to the incredible knowledge and smarts a heart surgeon possesses, coupled with the deft hands of some of the finest surgeons you will ever meet. I tried so very hard to resist its siren song, after each and every one of the consultant surgeons there lamented how much of their personal lives had been lost to the operating room.

CASE 3

The first day I went to the operating theatre in cardiac surgery, I was so nervous. I was scrubbing with the big boss, and he was known for wanting everything just so in his theatre. My job was to get to theatre, put on his favourite music, display the patient's X-ray on the screen and wait patiently for him. When he arrived, he barked, 'What are you waiting for? Go and get scrubbed.'

Under the watchful eye of the senior scrub nurse, I washed my hands. She ran a tight ship in the cardiac theatre, not just for her nurses but for the doctors as well, including the consultant surgeons. As we were scrubbing, she asked if I was ready. Ready for what, I wondered. 'They'll [referring to the consultants] give you a hard time. I hope you've got the balls to take it.'

Since I had been a medical student, I had become familiar with the penchant for hazing anyone new to the operating theatre. Most often, it was a ritual adhered to by the surgeons but, in reality, hazing could come from anyone. Some nurses would stop just shy of making you stand in the corner, like a dunce, lest you disrupt something you shouldn't. Anaesthetists would chuckle at any misfortune to befall you. And surgeons, well, some surgeons had a predictable formula for the jibes they would use to 'welcome' a new face to the fold.

If you were a man, you'd be teased about your ability, both good and bad. If you were unfamiliar with this skill or that procedure, someone would chuckle, 'Well, off to dermatology for you,' or any other specialty they deemed lesser, a place for washed-up surgical wannabes, offensive to that doctor and the specialty alike.

36

If you were a woman, you got teased about your ability too, but not before you'd have to listen to sexually inappropriate jokes. And if you weren't white, then it was ethnic (aka racist) jokes about your food, your name, the politics from your region. 'Don't worry, we'll be out of theatre soon enough so you can get back to your curry!' And finally, if you were the son or daughter of another doctor, then you'd also be teased for that. I was once told by a boss that it was to break the ice, but others have called it what it really was—totally inappropriate. I saw it as an opportunity to show how unshakable I was.

I took my place at the operating table as the boss surveyed me. He grabbed my hand in his, and placed it on the heart where I could feel it beating. It was magical, absolutely incredible. I could feel the power in each heartbeat but the fragility of it was not lost on me either. It just barely fitted into my hand; in between each forceful beat, the muscle softened and relaxed while the heart filled with blood before exploding with force again. The contraction pushed the blood out into the aorta where I could feel the whooshing past my hand. I had never seen anything like it before. I was in a daze, enamoured by this organ no bigger than my fist that kept this patient alive, when I was rudely interrupted by the boss saying, 'Now, since this is your first time scrubbing with me, if I "accidentally" grope you, I'm not sorry.'

'If you grope me,' I said, 'you'd better run,' making sure he could hear the jest in my voice, a feeble attempt to try to snap back, to prove that I was tough and completely unbothered by any hazing. I wasn't here to cause trouble; I just wanted to be a surgeon, no matter what. 'Ugh, you're not one of those bloody feminists, are you? Thinking that women can do anything that a man can do?'

Since I'd already poked the bear, I decided not to tell him that yes, I was a feminist and that yes, women can do anything a man can do. I carried on being smitten with the human heart, so much so that I did not care what was being said to me.

CRITICAL REFLECTION QUESTION
What do you observe about the life of a new RMO in this case study?

CASE 4
Nearly every day I'd stay at work long past going home time, sponging up as much as I could. I still came into work at 6 a.m. to do my obligatory paperwork with even more fervour than before so I could spend all day in theatre, learning how to be a heart surgeon. I was constantly in awe of what I thought was the crème de la crème of all medicine; I bathed in it every waking moment.

If cardiac surgery was the pinnacle of skill and knowledge, then transplantation was celestial. One of the first transplants I ever saw remains one of my favourite and most inspirational patients. Jenny was born with a congenital heart defect and was never expected to live past infancy. At the time she was born, heart surgery on children could still be a bit of a crapshoot. Some of the kids who underwent operations for complex heart defects they were unfortunate enough to be endowed with would die on the operating table, back when we lacked the knowledge or skills to repair their sick hearts. Rather than risk near-certain death with an operation, Jenny's heart had struggled through much of her life, damaging her lungs along the way and meaning that she needed a combined heart–lung transplant, one of the rarest transplants (fewer than ten of these operations would be performed in Australia most years).

I met her the morning of her surgery in the holding bay, a large, dimly lit room where bays filled with hospital trolleys (they're too primitive and uncomfortable to be called beds, even by hospital standards). Privacy is an illusion, inadequately provided by threadbare curtains around each bay in the open-plan room. I knew it was her from a mile away, her blue lips a giveaway as to her identity and her sick heart. She had waited so long for this moment, a call to say that someone had died so she could have a chance to live. We chatted and, looking back on this time now, I hope that my enthusiasm for seeing one of the rarest surgeries performed wasn't blatantly obvious in what was probably one of the most stressful times of her life.

When she eventually made her way through to the operating theatre, everything was already underway. In a distant operating theatre, another person was giving the ultimate

gift while she was being readied to face an enormous challenge. And thus began a surgery that took nearly twelve
hours. This was to be one of the most complex surgeries
I had ever seen, the complexity compounded by how sick this
brave woman was and her highly complicated and unusual
heart defect. On the floor in the operating theatre, empty
bags of donated blood begun to pile up to catalogue their
use. The room was constantly abuzz, with a team of dozens
of doctors, nurses and other specialist staff working and
learning simultaneously. As if the pressure wasn't already
high, in the midst of the surgery, a power failure caused
a moment of panic; the life-sustaining heart–lung bypass
machine obviously depends on electricity and in the event
of a power failure, the machine must be hand-cranked by as
many people as possible.

Thankfully, the back-up generators kicked in and
the operation finally concluded as night began to fall. As the
surgical drapes were removed, the results of the successful
operation were evident not only on the monitor, with the
new heart and lungs easily maintaining life unassisted, but
in the changed colour of her lips. Once blue, her lips were
now a very normal and very reassuring shade of pink. Later
on, back in the intensive care unit, her mother would remark
with great joy how it was the first time she had ever seen her
daughter with pink lips, the blueness banished.

While the surgery was phenomenal, the aftermath was
a long and hard road to recovery. A series of complications slowed her recovery but, day by day, she got stronger,

defeating each obstacle placed in her way to make a full recovery. What a privilege it was to witness that tenacity and eventual triumph to the day when she finally walked out of the hospital, liberated from the depressing hospital ward. Even as fascinating and challenging as the surgery was, what really got me was that someone had a second chance at life. How could I not want to help deliver that gift to as many people as possible? The pride and sense of wonderment that she brought me lingers on today, as if I was still there, in her hospital room, all those years ago.

CRITICAL REFLECTION QUESTION
What do you observe about the life of a new RMO in this case study?

Not long after that marathon surgery came the clincher that would ensure I was ensnared by cardiothoracic surgery forever. It was another transplant patient, this time a man who was having a lung transplant. In comparison to the previous lady, there wasn't nearly as much fanfare, with this being a 'run of the mill' lung transplant, as run of the mill as a lung transplant can be.

Lung transplants fascinated me then. Most of the time, we perform lung transplants on both sides, termed bilaterally, in a sequential fashion and, at the time, we did them without the aid of a heart–lung bypass machine. Once inside the rib cage, the most diseased lung is freed from its roots by dividing the bronchus (the extension of the windpipe that carries air), the pulmonary artery (the big blood vessel that delivers oxygen-poor blood to the lungs for replenishment) and finally the pulmonary veins, which carry oxygen-rich blood back to the heart for distribution to the rest of our body. One side of the chest is then empty, leaving a cavernous space with the ribs on display. The new lung is sewn into its new home and, like virtually all transplanted organs, once it's connected to its new blood supply it just starts working.

While the new lung settles in, we turn our attention to the other side where the remaining diseased lung is also removed and replaced by the new lung in the exact same way. And in the exact same way as the previous side, it too just knows its role, immediately getting on with the job of taking in vital oxygen and dispelling carbon dioxide. And for this man, who had depended on an oxygen cylinder being wheeled behind him all the time, that is exactly how it went. As is so often in surgery, what was uneventful for us surgeons was the most enormous event for him and his family.

A couple of days after his surgery, on the ward round, he looked so healthy and happy it was almost as though nothing had happened. The only evidence of the surgery were the remnant tubes and connections that come complimentary with a major surgery. I stood by his bedside and asked him what I thought was the most banal question: 'How are you going?'

He looked me dead in the eye and replied, 'You have no idea how good it feels to be able to breathe.'

I was sold. Right then and there, my stubborn pursuit of my original dream of a career in orthopaedics was finally erased by his words. How could I ever turn away from a career where I might be able to give patients the simple yet vital gift of breathing?

I had to admit defeat, which involved going with my tail between my legs to my consultants and telling them that I had indeed been bewitched by cardiac surgery and that was what I was going to chase down with all of my ambition. Despite my previous protestations that I would never be attracted to cardiothoracics the same way that I was interested in fixing people's bones and joints, it turned out my resistance was futile and my eight-year-old self had known far better.

Somewhat cruelly, my term in cardiothoracics came to an end and I was off to my next rotation, in orthopaedics. There, the love was most definitely gone, like a summer crush forgotten on the first day of school. My heart was not in it anymore and, while the science and art of repairing bones was interesting, it lacked the frisson that cardiac surgery had brought me. It was going to be a long three months in my orthopaedic rotation because I wanted to be somewhere else altogether.

* * *

43

Part of the selection process to get into medical school involved an interview designed to find, I assume, those who would be our most gifted healers. I practised questions on ethics and teamwork with no problem. But the question I feared the most was why I wanted to be a doctor. I couldn't think of a way to explain how it just felt right, like my soul was set on fire at the idea of helping people.

It felt a little the same for cardiothoracic surgery. Something about it just lit me up inside with a passion that I couldn't quite articulate. When you love something so deeply, it can be hard to explain exactly why it is that you're so drawn to it, except to say that you are. And for me, I could trace that passion back to my childhood, when I used to raid the library for books on how the human body worked and imagine stepping in and saving a life before I was even old enough to properly understand what exactly that meant.

The heart is remarkable. I am obviously incredibly biased but I think that it is just the most fascinating thing. It starts beating when the embryo is only four weeks old and unless someone like me interferes with it, it never stops, not until the day you die. My favourite thing about the heart is that the muscle cells that make it up are autonomous. All they need is fresh, oxygenated blood and they just know to contract. And when they all contract in a perfectly choreographed rhythm, the heart beats.

Seeing and holding a human heart was just an indescribable feeling. During surgery, when you place your hand on it, you can feel every heartbeat and how each rhythmical squeeze of the heart changes with each little thing we do—it reacts and changes with the blood we infuse, with medications. When the operation is completed, you can see an immediate change in the heart's function as it is relieved of the ailment that brought it there in the first place.

It wasn't just the heart and how remarkable it is that made me fall in love. As much as I was fascinated by every little part of the heart and how it worked, I was equally in awe of the people I worked with. Cardiac surgery felt different to my time in other specialties in the way that an enormous team of people come together and work so closely with each other all for one greater good: the patient.

From the beginning to the end of the patient's journey, they will be taken care of by dozens of different doctors, nurses, physiotherapists, medical scientists: you name it. And, back then at least, the cohesiveness of this team was just remarkable to me. In the operating theatre alone, there were two anaesthetists, an anaesthetic registrar and anaesthetic nurse, a consultant surgeon, two or three surgical registrars, a scrub nurse and a circulating nurse who gets equipment as we need it. And, of course, a perfusionist, the scientist who runs the heart–lung bypass machine. Which means on most days a single patient could have at least ten people overseeing their stay in the operating theatre.

It was never the sheer number of people present—though that was remarkable to me: it was the way they all worked together. I'd never seen anything like it before—everyone brought a special set of skills to the table and worked in concert and harmony. In the rest of the hospital, we all inter-mingle to a degree but I cannot think of another team so enmeshed with each other like this. Not only was the team numerous, they also seemed to function with a genuine care for each other and for the work they did. This team that I started out with would go on to be my team for most of my career; they would become my confidants, my friends, all bound together by the fact that we loved what we did and we respected the people that we did it with.

I used to look at the consultants in cardiothoracics in complete awe. In my mind, they were about as close to gods, to superheroes, as one could possibly be. I admired just about everything they did, from their extraordinary medical knowledge, the deftness of their hands and the way they seemed to dedicate themselves totally and utterly to their role, often supported by their girlfriends, ex-wives and paid assistants. These men became my mentors and friends; I wanted to spend as much time as I could with them, purely to lap up their greatness.

One of my bosses stood out in particular. I loved the way he commanded a room, everyone listening to every word, I thought purely by virtue of his incredible skill. He was young, recently divorced and lived alone like a tortured artist wholly dedicated to his craft. Over the years we grew close, as mentor and mentee. One day, we were at his house and he asked me out on a date, which I flatly refused. My declining didn't stop him from trying to kiss me as I left his house. I should never have been there in the first place, and he should never have done that but I was so taken with his skills as a surgeon I had pushed my discomfort down as far as it would go.

Although I was forgiving, I wasn't completely ignorant to his and the other consultants' shortcomings; I saw the trail of broken relationships and tenuous connections with their children for some of them. I felt the sting of shitty, inappropriate jokes and temper tantrums in operating theatres. But I didn't care. I saw all the personal sacrifice as a marker of how dedicated they were to their jobs, as a kind of medal of valour, and the unprofessional slips in behaviour as either excusable in light of their greatness or understandable given what they were responsible for.

But I think the most remarkable thing for me was the patients. They were incredibly brave, of course, but I was mostly struck by how dramatically their lives could be changed by what we could do: how they could go from not being able to breathe, being incapable of doing even the simplest things like getting dressed, even quite literally being at death's door, to having a chance at life. In the space of hours, we could wrestle them from disease and suffering and put them on a path of living a normal, or at least vastly improved, life. This wasn't me measuring my greatness by how positively I could affect someone else's life; it was a deep emotional response to seeing someone have their hopes realised. I didn't need it to necessarily be me delivering that hope, delivering health. I loved just being a small part of the team who made that happen. What I truly lived for was knowing that, even in the direst of circumstances, people could be helped; people could even be saved.

One thing I came to realise about heart surgery is that you have to love it. Some would say you have to love it more than anything else in your life. More than your spouse, your children, your hobbies. Even more than yourself. When I finally built up enough courage to tell one of my bosses that I thought I wanted to do cardiothoracics, he looked at me and said, 'I hope you're willing to give up everything. Because that's what you'll have to do.'

He explained to me that cardiac surgery was different and unique. When the phone rings at 2 a.m., you can't whinge and complain how you hate it. You have to be completely and utterly enamoured to get out of bed and be the best you can possibly be because somebody's life depends on it. A transplant won't wait because it's your wedding anniversary or your daughter's birthday. Your run and your doctor's appointment will always take a backseat, because when you stop loving cardiac surgery, the risk is that it will show in your work. Cardiac surgery is, and will always have to be, your one true love. No matter what.

Far from deterring me, this only confirmed what I already knew. I was completely, totally and utterly in love with the heart. And the only thing I wanted was to be a heart surgeon. I started to realise that I couldn't picture my life with anything else. I didn't care about sacrifice; I didn't care that it would be hard and challenging. I saw nothing else except reaching that goal. Even though I was cautioned, it wasn't stubbornness that made me disregard that message. It was blind love for what I wanted to do. What could possibly go wrong if you adored what you did? That's what you're told, isn't it? If you do something you love, you'll never work a day in your life? For me, passion above all else was the most important thing when it came to choosing a career.

For the most part, that love never went away. To this day, I can still be completely floored by the heart, by the team and by the patients. When the operation is complete and the heart just starts working again, that sight never stops being remarkable. When the sick heart is suddenly better because of something that we've done, that is still an extraordinary gift. When the team rallies together to save a life, it still warms my soul with so much gratitude to be a part of it.

That's the thing about all-consuming blind love. No matter what goes on around you, whether you should have noticed it or not, a love like that will always be a part of you, will always set your soul on fire and will lead you to do just about anything for it. Whether you should or not is a different question altogether.

3

JUNIOR REGISTRAR
Still in the shit

I still remember the first surgery I ever performed solo, long before I was captivated by the heart. I was just an intern, rotating through general surgery, and the first operation I ever did myself was to drain a peri-anal abscess: an abscess that forms near the anus and is incredibly painful for the patient, thus, I was a hero despite the fact that the operation took all of about ten minutes.

After finishing, I wrote up the operation report, where the surgeon records details of what they've just done so that it's preserved for all eternity. It's the piece of paper that explains where the incision was made, what was found and what was done. And it's also where you record who actually did the operation. I was so pleased to be able to write 'Surgeon: Stamp' for the first time, which, looking back on that now, is both endearing and the dorkiest thing I've probably done.

I often feel like a surgical career is marked by firsts. The first operation you ever did, the first operation you did solo, the first amazing save you made, the first time on call and so on, throughout your career. Incidentally, the first ever operation I saw was an orchidectomy, which is the surgical removal of a testicle and I thought it was fascinating.

Even though I had completely sold my soul to cardiac surgery, giddy with the heart and everyone who helped to mend it, now that I had graduated from RMO to service registrar, I had to spend time in other surgical specialties. All of which I treated with a sense of pity that that specialty, in my mind, would never be as sexy as heart surgery. Sexy was how one of my bosses described heart surgery, as in it's 'sexy, doc, chicks dig it'. It was certainly attractive to me, perhaps not in the way he meant.

To make sure we all got a good breadth of experience, even once we were hopelessly dedicated to our one true love, registrars had to rotate through the various surgical specialities—I threw myself into every specialty, trying to sponge up every bit of knowledge that I could, do as much operating as I could and even sometimes 'try on' that specialty to see if it was going to be something I would be able to do for the rest of my career. But on weekends, or days off, I'd cheat on that specialty with cardiothoracics, assisting my bosses doing cases in private hospitals just so I could get my fix of hearts.

Most of my time during those years were spent in general surgery, probably the oldest surgical specialty there is.

General surgery is predominantly concerned with the abdomen, the bowel, the stomach and the liver but also the breast and some of the endocrine (hormone) organs like the thyroid. General surgery is where I have met some of the finest surgeons, whose breadth of experience, skill and knowledge is deeply impressive. One of the first major surgeries I ever scrubbed in for was an oesophagectomy—the removal of virtually the entire oesophagus, the tube that connects your mouth to your stomach—for cancer. I was so enamoured of the enormity of the operation, the anatomy, the seeming heroics of the surgeons, that I thought I might want to be an upper GI surgeon. These surgeons put their undies on the outside every day to tackle the complexities of the top part of the gastrointestinal tract: the oesophagus, the stomach and the pancreas. This is tiger country for surgeons, requiring an extraordinary amount of bravery, skill and perhaps insanity in equal measures. The oesophagectomies would have to tide me over during my time as the general surgery registrar, keeping me in my spiritual home in the chest.

But I was about to discover that being the general surgery registrar is one of the toughest gigs in the hospital. It's probably the busiest surgical services, taking care of people with belly pain, appendicitis and people who have been involved in serious traumas. When you're on call, your pager or phone virtually never stops ringing with referrals from the emergency department or questions from other inpatient teams. Most of my days on call in general surgery

I was so busy I didn't have time to eat or even pee, which wasn't an issue because I had no time to drink water either. Most doctors are more dehydrated than their patients. Sometimes I'd have two or three phones on the go at once, juggling two or three different problems.

From the emergency department, virtually anyone who turns up with some form of pain in their abdomen will be reviewed by the general surgery registrar on call. You would go down to the ED, which was inevitably heaving with patients in every nook and cranny. You'd have to try to find somewhere quiet and private to examine them, so as not to expose them to the entire corridor where they had been parked for hours, awaiting an answer to whatever had brought them in. Moving the beds around in ED was kind of like Tetris, trying to work out whom you could fit in where.

The fact that general surgery is largely concerned with the guts means that there is a strange obsession with people's poo. Virtually every patient, every morning on the ward round, is asked, in more detail than is normally considered polite conversation, about their bowel movements, including if they'd 'passed wind' (a refined way of enquiring about someone's farts). Virtually nothing was off limits in the world of general surgery. Given that in general surgery we were often dealing with people's most rarely spoken about body parts and functions, an immunity to embarrassment was essential. Nobody wants to see their doctor turn bright red when trying to detail something about their bowel movements or, sometimes, things that were even more personal.

Despite the fact that I was wholly dedicated to life as a heart surgeon, I actually enjoyed general surgery. I enjoyed the breadth of cases I was involved in, the business of the job and working with some of the best surgeons, who were also among the kindest and most magnificent teachers that I had ever worked with. And general surgery was well known for giving what we called 'cutting time'—what every surgical wannabe lives for. It's a crude way of describing getting the opportunity to actually do some operating, rather than just assisting or watching. Basically, for those of us desperate to advance in our career in surgery, we just want to operate. We jostle and plan to make sure that, when that first incision is made on the patient, the scalpel is in our hand. Sometimes we hip and shoulder our way into cases ahead of our colleagues. Other times we beg and negotiate with our bosses and even with our fellow registrars because 'I've never seen one of these before!' or 'I admitted this patient and I really want to be there with them'. Whatever the reason, the more operating, the better. It was all about getting those all-important opportunities to show what you've learnt, to demonstrate to your boss just how well you could whip out an appendix and, maybe, get given the opportunity to be taught something more.

The more time you were there, the more you got to do. You might start with an appendix and then, as you proved yourself, you took on more complex cases. Some of the battle was showing you had the skills to do the procedure, but a lot of it was showing that you had the balls. The courage to jostle your way to the operating table, to stay up late into the night, to impress your boss and basically to be tough enough to survive the baptism of fire. Then your reward was operating. And what a reward it was. Slowly but surely, I saw my logbook of surgical cases grow and grow. I stared at the numbers of procedures I had under my belt with enormous pride.

CASE 5

It was a typically busy on-call, the usually twenty-four hour period of being the general surgery doctor, who would be notified of anything that might need the skills of the general surgery service. I met a man who had been sent from another hospital after having had a colonoscopy. A colonoscopy is a test where you get a little medicine to let you lightly sleep and the doctor puts a camera up the backside and looks at the bowel. It's a really common test and is often done to look for bowel cancer. This gentleman likely had bowel cancer: he'd barely gone to the toilet for nearly six weeks, he told me. To prepare the bowel for the colonoscopy, patients drink a few litres of a drink called bowel prep, which basically induces diarrhoea to empty the bowel so that the doctor doing the scope has an unimpeded view.

The problem for this man was that it turned out that the reason he hadn't had a poo for so long was that he did indeed have a bowel cancer that had grown so large it was basically obstructing his bowel. When the camera was put in, the pressure caused a little tear in the bowel, which is incredibly dangerous. The inside of our bowel is filled with bacteria, which is generally beneficial, but when it makes its way outside our bowel into the abdominal cavity, it causes a life-threatening infection called peritonitis. Peritonitis is a genuine medical emergency. And that was the precarious situation this lovely man found himself in. What was supposed to have been a short procedure to give him an answer and have him home before evening had taken a turn to become a genuinely life-threatening problem.

It was off to the operating theatre for emergency surgery. My boss began the operation, expertly opening the abdomen with a cut right down the middle of the belly. He dove into the abdomen, delivering the bowel to the outside world and quickly identifying the big lump in the bowel that would turn out to be bowel cancer. The only way to deal with this as well as the tear in the bowel was to cut out that section of the bowel. The bowel is like a tube, so when you cut one part out you have to rejoin the two ends. In the bad old days of surgery, surgeons would hand-sew the two cut ends of the bowel back together. But in modern times, we have staplers that quickly and effectively do that for us, enabling a faster, more secure join. One side of the stapler was fired from inside the abdomen, and the other side was fired by someone who sat between the patient's legs: that person is usually the most junior doctor who, today, was me.

I dutifully took my place on a stool and gently inserted the stapler into the patient's rectum and readied myself to pull the trigger on the boss's instruction. He divided the last of the bowel as we fired our respective staplers. And with that, six weeks' worth of shit fell on to my lap and into my white hospital-issued gumboots. Despite the uncomfortable nature of this situation, you can't necessarily run off for a shower. But, on that day, my boss was kind enough to let me go, replacing me with another registrar so that I could shower and change my scrubs.

My only thought at that moment was, 'Please, get me back to the chest'.

CRITICAL REFLECTION QUESTION
What do you observe about the life of a registrar in this case study? How would you approach this situation?

I didn't have to wait long to return to cardiothoracics; in just a few weeks I would be rotating back to a place where the only thing I could be covered in was blood. For my obsession with all things heart, I was about to be handsomely rewarded. That was the norm: education was not seen as a right for junior doctors but rather as a prize to be earned. And, perhaps through my enthusiasm, I had earned a shot at putting a patient on to bypass, which meant that my own heart was aflutter with excitement.

When we perform heart surgery, we have to connect the patient to the heart–lung machine. The cardiopulmonary bypass machine revolutionised heart surgery; it allowed us to stop the heart and see inside it, repair it and restart it. Before its advent, surgeons couldn't operate or, sometimes, would have to make a hole in the heart while it was still beating, and sew up whatever defect they were battling against quickly before the patient bled to death. Heart surgeons even used to join a child needing heart surgery to their parent through a series of tubes called cross-circulation, where the parent's circulation would act as the heart–lung machine. But now we have a big, shiny machine that safely does all of this, under the watchful eye of a perfusionist, a highly skilled member of the team who controls almost every aspect of the patient's physiology during the heart surgery.

Connecting someone to this machine isn't straightforward. Going on to bypass is a critical moment in the surgery. It's kind of like taking off and landing an aircraft: the lights are dimmed and everyone is strapped in safely because it's a moment when things can go wrong. That day, I was about to, for the first time, pilot that take-off by connecting someone to the heart–lung bypass machine; since it was so critical, it had to be a smooth take-off.

My boss stood opposite me, gently directing me through the process. The heart sat on display and I started the process. To hold in the pipes that make the connection, I placed sutures in a circle that would act as a purse string, snugly holding the pipes inside the heart. I can still remember how my hands shook as I took the shiny needle holder, an instrument that looked a bit like scissors, and used them to guide the semicircular needle to gently place the stitch in the aorta, followed by one in the right atrium in preparation for me to introduce massive pipes into the heart.

With my purse strings in place, the actual scary part was next. I had to plunge a scalpel blade into the aorta, making a hole to slide in the cannula, a pipe about the size of my index finger. It has to be done quickly and smoothly, because around five litres of blood a minute rushes out at a speed of two to three metres per second, which means that, through this relatively small hole, it's possible for blood to not only hit the ceiling (I've seen that happen) but also for the patient's entire blood volume to be out of their body in around five minutes flat.

It's hard to fight against the logical part of your brain that rightly tells you that making holes in the heart is a bad thing (which is where I assume my shaking was coming from). Shaking hands do not make for a smooth take-off, which my boss reminded me. I took a second to take a big breath, relax my shoulders and forget that I could decorate the ceiling with blood if I screwed this up. But the most calming thing was that my boss said to me, 'I wouldn't let you do this if I thought you couldn't. But more importantly, I wouldn't let you do it if I didn't know I could fix any problem that you make. Because, trust me, I've seen them all.'

The shake steadied just enough and I took the scalpel and made a hole inside the circle of my suture in the aorta and then quickly slid the cannula into place. I'd like to say it wasn't messy but it was a little untidy, unlike when I do it now when I aim to let barely a single red cell escape. I then repeated this process in the right atrium, sliding in a bigger pipe that would take blood from the heart to the machine to be cleansed, oxygenated and returned to the patient via the cannula in the aorta. With all the tubing connected, I said to the perfusionist, 'Go on to bypass, thanks', and watched the blood start to drain away from the right atrium and the heart deflate like a balloon emptying, only to return, pristine, to the aorta, sustaining life.

My boss said to me, 'Nicely done, now go and finish sewing up the leg,' from where I had just harvested a vein.

My nerves turned to elation, as I mentally added 'Putting someone on bypass' to my list of firsts in surgery. And what a first! It felt like 'real' heart surgery, not just stealing veins from legs and sewing up wounds. Even though all of these things are truly important to an operation going smoothly, they don't feel as exciting as getting to operate on the actual heart. For the rest of the case I was positively buzzing, beaming beneath my mask while the patient remained asleep, blissfully unaware that they were my first serious foray into actually being a heart surgeon.

The patient was taken to the ICU after his surgery and I stood at his bedside, ready to add his details to my logbook. I was thrilled but also intent on seeing that everything was fine. I studied his vitals intently. Even though I had only done one small portion of the surgery, in my mind, it was massive. And I wanted to make sure that the patient's contribution to this momentous point in my life was as rewarding for him as it was for me, with a safe and speedy recovery.

Two days later, he was out of the intensive care unit, back on our normal ward, sitting up eating breakfast while we did our ward round, almost as if nothing had happened. As if two days earlier we hadn't been tinkering with his heart. I could feel a weight lift as the team of doctors and nurses on the ward round all noted how everything was going according to plan.

As we checked the wounds on his leg and his chest, both of which I had sewn up with the utmost of care, he said to the room, 'Who is your seamstress? Bloody good job they've done here!' and I grinned from ear to ear but kept quiet in the gaggle. Our senior registrar just thanked him for his compliment and reassured him that he was well on his way to recovery.

But in my head, I silently thanked him for his invaluable contribution on my journey to being a surgeon.

* * *

I tend to talk a lot about how much I love the science of medicine. How I could spend all day and all night elbows deep in every little detail of the human body and how it works. Or studying disease intently so I could 'know my enemy' in order to defeat it.

Even as a medical student, I simply could not learn enough. Only a few years into medical school, I was browsing through a secondhand bookshop when I came across a book of surgical instruments. I clutched it tight to my chest, ignoring the other offerings on the shelves to buy it before anyone else could. Which is adorable: I thought I was going to have to fight off a crowd for this very niche book.

The pages were filled with pictures of shiny instruments, some for cutting, others for sewing. There were entire chapters dedicated to instruments that held tissue back, called retractors, and an endless array of needle holders, each with tiny differences that made them particularly good at whatever job they were intended for. Under each picture was its name: Castroviejo needle holders, Langenbeck retractors, Metzenbaum scissors and Cooley clamps, all named for great men of surgery. I wondered what one had to do to have an instrument named after them and added it to my mental list of career goals.

Surgery isn't just about being book smart though. I absolutely adored learning the skills of surgery. One of the skills I most wanted to acquire early on was something we call hand-tying. A surgeon's knots are some of the most important things they can do, with sutures tied inside the human body responsible for holding together the most fragile or the most important tissues. 'Do you trust your knots?' my favourite old surgeon would ask me, leading me to wonder if I would lie awake at night in a cold sweat, hoping that my knots could withstand the pressure of pulsating blood.

In med school, while I was memorising instruments named for obscure European doctors from days gone by, I was also practising my hand-ties. When it's done well, a hand-tie looks a little like a magician casting a spell; the fingers do a beautiful little dance around each other and the suture and all of a sudden, presto! A perfectly laid square knot that will save a life. I used to practise my hand-ties at any opportunity with virtually every doorknob in my house, making what seemed like kilometres of perfectly neat and robust rows of knots. As I worked to get my hands to dance in the same perfect way my consultants' hands did, I found just sitting around tying knots upon knots to be a kind of relaxing thing to do, like I had found my happy place.

All of this was done to be perfect. After all, as I was told time and time again, in cardiac surgery our motto was 'Near enough is not good enough'. We needed to be exceptional in every aspect of everything that we did. This suited me just fine, because I loved what I was doing so much I wanted to know everything and be able to do everything. I wanted to be perfect in everything that I did out of passion.

At the start of my surgical career, being good was all about wanting to excel at the thing that made me tick. And if I'm honest, there was also a healthy dose of just wanting to be the best at it too. With more and more time in the hospitals, away from textbooks and door handles, more and more I wanted to be good for another, incredibly important reason.

When you're learning in the operating theatre and the boss is yelling at you or pushing you to be better, it's easy to forget that you're not doing it for him (it would be nearly ten years after I left medical school before I would work for a boss who was a 'her'). Sometimes in surgery we get carried away, thinking that we're trying to impress the boss or, for the ultra-competitive among us, trying to outdo each other. In reality, adages like 'close enough is not good enough' are there for a far greater reason: for the patients.

* * *

It wasn't something that had truly sunk in for me until I started doing more and more on patients. With every stitch I placed in living human flesh, the understanding that someone was relying on me to be flawless became less of a cognitive awareness and more of something I felt in my soul. The more patients I saw on the ward round after operations where I had done some or all of the procedure, the more I truly understood what was at stake.

While the science of surgery fascinated and stimulated me, the patients are the ones who made me want to get out of bed every day. From medical school, with each passing year, the more people I spoke to, cared for and operated on, the more I wanted to be the best not just for myself or the love of what I was doing, but for them. I owed it to my patients to be exceptional since they were quite literally placing their lives in my hands.

The importance of this was never more acute than when I was learning. The odd thing about surgery is that no matter how much practice you've had tying knots on strings, studying textbooks or observing your boss, you will always have to do something for the first time on a real patient, a person who has hopes and dreams and an astonishing amount of trust in us, their doctors, to not just do the best that they can. They need us to be as close to perfect as we can possibly be.

As a registrar, knowing that someone is trusting you to learn on them when they are at their most vulnerable is a strange feeling to have, even at times a burden to carry. There are so many patients who served as firsts for me, but they don't stand out to me just because they represent the transition from practising skills on a piece of string or studying textbooks all night. They were real people who were someone's loved one and that mattered even more than a new skill that I learnt. I remember so many of these people who were firsts so clearly, their stories imprinted on my mind forever.

I loved talking to patients, hearing their stories and knowing who they were and where they came from. The more I got to know them, the more I wanted everything to go well for them. Medicine still has this idea that doctors should keep a distance from their patients, lest we get too emotional and involved in their care and it clouds our judgement. But I couldn't turn away from getting to know that person and caring about them, not just as a chance for me to do a procedure I hadn't done yet or as a bed number on a chart. The more I cared about them, the more I wanted to be better at what I did so that I could make sure they went home safely.

As I started to learn more about surgery, I began to understand the great service that these people were doing. The first time I went to put in a chest drain, a small tube about the size of your finger to drain fluid from around the lung, the patient asked me how many of these I had done before. My senior registrar looked about as nervous as I felt to answer the question.

'Just one,' I told him, because I'm a terrible liar. I doubt I could have found the bravado to say anything else. My senior jumped in and hurriedly assured the patient that he had done many hundreds and would be with me all the way. I half-expected this man, whose breathing was laboured and uncomfortable from the fluid around his left lung, to say that he'd sooner keep suffocating than let me notch up chest drain number two on him. But he didn't.

'Well, I suppose you have to learn somehow.' And with that, I was filled with gratitude. Because he was absolutely correct. I did have to learn somehow and inevitably, it was going to be on him.

The more I got to do on real people, and the more I got to see the results of my handiwork, the more my motivation to be great started to be driven by a much more important, moral imperative. The drive to do right by that patient was the reason for knots on door handles and being glued to textbooks. It was a reason I knew I could endure a decade of training, with long nights, isolation and stress that many people would never know in their careers. It would be the reason I would look at my own suturing with a critical eye, knowing that the next day on the ward, I'd have to look that person in the eye and tell them that I had done a good job, even a great one.

4

TRAINEE REGISTRAR

It *is* heart surgery

'What interests you in cardiothoracic surgery?'

'I find the surgery fascinating and I really like helping people and I . . . I think the heart is so fascinating.'

I stared in the mirror, exasperated with myself. Come on, Nikki, you have done better than this. Focus and answer the damn question.

I had travelled to Melbourne for the second year in a row with my partner, who was training to be an emergency physician, to interview for a position on the cardiothoracic surgery training program. The year before, I had had my own heart broken when I missed out on the prestigious program by just a few positions in the ranking. In all honesty, I knew that it was probably too soon and another year as a service registrar (a non-training position that feels a little like limbo) would only add to my experience and my maturity. But I had cried my eyes out nonetheless, devastated to have to face the reality that just wanting it badly wasn't enough.

As I got dressed, I was trying to stay focused on all of the interview questions I had practised so that I knew I was bringing my A game. I was worried that I may have chosen to wear too feminine an outfit to be interviewed for a position in a specialty that had only eight women in its ranks at that stage. And I was haunted by my devastation from the year before of not making it.

All of my eggs were in this one surgical basket.

In Australia, to become a specialist in anything, you have to be accepted into and complete a training program. It is similar to an apprenticeship, if that apprenticeship involved sleep deprivation, expensive training fees and more study than you had ever done before in your life. All while trying to keep other humans alive. While you're working towards being welcomed into the brethren of surgical trainees, you mark time as a service or unaccredited registrar: a cannon fodder, mid-level doctor who is supposed to be on their way to a training position—but for some that position never eventuates. Partly because it's in the best interests of those in power and those footing the bill to have a captive audience of mid-level doctors paid less, for their apparent inexperience, to do a huge amount of hard work, enticed by the possibility of their career dreams. It's simultaneously demoralising and a waste of their time and our taxpayer money. I didn't know it at the time but medicine, and surgery in particular, are pyramid schemes, only ever allowing a select few to make it to the top.

That year, cardiothoracic surgery was taking just three young hopefuls from Australia and New Zealand. It must seem puzzling, given that the news is regularly telling us how we have shortages of doctors and specialists. Training positions are rare because in some ways they have to be—training a specialist is expensive and labour intensive and there literally is not enough time and space for everyone. Not to mention that at the end of that training we need to employ them as consultants, and we definitely don't manage that—many surgeons may be unable to find such a job. Plus, if I'm cynical (which I am), I can't discount that keeping us in a perpetual state of supposed insignificance protects the power and the money for those at the top of the ladder. It's a complex and frustrating system that today, even after nearly two decades of mulling it over, I'm yet to arrive at a satisfactory explanation or an alternative to.

Out of dozens of applicants, the odds were not in anyone's favour for a paltry three places. But I had learnt from last year's stumble and come back a stronger, better applicant; it was basically now or never.

'Thank you for coming, Dr Stamp. We'll start with an easy one. Why do you want to be a cardiothoracic surgeon?'

I smiled at the interviewer. Good start, a question I had practised.

CASE 6
'Give it to the boy.'

That was me, the boy. My boss used to call all of his junior staff his 'boy'. Occasionally, he'd call me the girl, but

I responded to both. I suppose he did so to infantilise us, to demonstrate his position as the patriarch of the unit, but, although he claimed to use it as a term of endearment, he seemed to fail to understand the horrific racist connotations that really should have stopped him from ever saying this.

Just a year earlier, I had gotten a phone call that had changed my life, telling me that, in all of Australia and New Zealand, I was one of the three doctors who was going to go on to be a cardiothoracic surgeon that year. Which meant at this hospital, I was heir to the title of 'the boy' and sometimes the novel title, the girl.

It was my first few weeks back in cardiothoracic surgery as the trainee, after spending a year rotating through other specialties to broaden my experience. There is a chasm of expectations between being a trainee, someone who has dedicated their life to training and working in that specialty, and being a service registrar, someone just passing through. All of a sudden, the responsibilities increase exponentially, as do the expectations of your knowledge and time that you're expected to give to your job.

Although I felt ready and willing to disregard everything else in my life, I had somehow squeezed in time to marry a fellow doctor, my emergency medicine registrar boyfriend. I used to love the fact that as someone going through the same system I was, he would fully understand the dedication to my job. However, unlike the cruelty of surgery, emergency medicine seemed to give a shit about their trainees. And he never fully understood why I had to and wanted to sell my soul for this job.

I was standing opposite my boss, helping him to perform an aortic valve replacement. The aortic valve is the main blood vessel out of the heart, and the biggest artery in the body, taking blood around the entire circulatory system. It has a valve at the bottom of it, just at the exit from the heart, to keep blood heading in the right direction. Disease of this valve is very common, meaning it needs to be replaced to stop the heart from eventually failing.

To perform this surgery, the heart is connected to the heart–lung bypass machine to make an incision as long as five centimetres in the aorta to pull out the diseased valve (it goes in the bin) and replace it with a new valve, made from the valve of a pig—the technical term for this is a 'porcine bioprosthesis'. The hole in the aorta obviously needs to be closed and, just like it was done in the early days of heart surgery, it has to be hand-sewn. No machines or staplers here.

My boss had closed the side closest to him when he instructed the scrub nurse to give me (aka the boy) the needle holder and the blue thread to continue the closure. This is how heart surgery is taught: in dribs and drabs, until eventually the dribs and drabs add up to a whole operation you do entirely yourself. I'd never done this before, but I had of course seen it countless times. I was beyond excited to be sewing up a real-life heart, because, in those early days, all of the small things you get to do for the first time are exciting. In my mind, I was just a short step away from basically doing the whole thing myself.

The boss and the anaesthetist worked with the perfusionist to slowly wake up the heart and separate the patient from the heart–lung bypass machine. A clamp is taken off the aorta, above where we made the cut to access the old valve, and blood rushes back to the heart. My favourite thing about the heart is that, when you give the heart muscle cells oxygen-rich blood, the heart just starts beating, usually without encouragement. And that is exactly what happened, meaning that the pipes in the heart could be safely removed.

Once that was done, my boss left me to close the patient. This is probably the least exciting part of the operation and, in theory, the most straightforward, so it's often left to the trainee and is totally safe to do so. He always told me where he would be; sometimes that was in the theatre in the corner on the phone, or in the office outside, just a few moments away. Today, it was a little further afield, but I knew I was capable and safe to finish the case.

Two things that are an absolute necessity before restoring the chest to something that resembles normal is that the heart is beating happily and there is no bleeding. As I started to sew closed the pericardium, the fibrous sac that the heart normally sits in, there was a bit too much blood for my liking. So I re-opened the pericardium and saw a tiny hole on the surface of the heart, in the right ventricle. I told the anaesthetist that I just needed to quickly stitch the hole closed and it shouldn't be a problem. But my inexperience was going to cause a problem bigger than the one I had just found.

The right ventricle is thin-walled, responsible for pumping blood under low pressure to the lungs. Because of this, it's a little more fragile than its cousin on the left side, which is thick and muscular to be able to cope with the demands of the entire body. This meant that, as my needle plunged into the right ventricle, the hole that had been only a few milli-metres to begin with all of a sudden became large enough for me to put my thumb in.

I was the most senior surgeon in the room then, so I needed to take action. I got the perfusionist and the heart–lung machine back in the room; the anaesthetist was busy organising blood to transfuse and the scrub nurses (who are heroes in dire situations like this) were getting all of the things I needed to go back on to bypass. All while my finger was plugging the hole in the bucket. And, of course, I asked someone to get the boss—'Someone find him and get him back here right now!'

This was the first time I had ever had to crash back on to bypass (another first). And I had to do it with blood pouring out and a hole in the right ventricle that seemed to keep enlarging (it was). But it took just a few minutes to have the machine back in charge and I could then see the damage clearly. At that moment, the boss poked his head into the door at the side of theatre, and he wasn't wearing scrubs. When he inquired what was going on, I think I was a little terse when my response was that he had better be getting changed and getting back in here now.

This boss was always my favourite to have around when something went wrong (and he still is). He once told me that there isn't much he hasn't seen and that was evident in situations like this. He didn't push me aside, but rather guided me to learn how to fix problems myself. He coached me as I sewed a patch over the hole in the heart (we still had no idea what had caused the original hole) and once again separated man from machine and closed the chest safely.

As he left, one of the anaesthetists thanked him for coming back to help, to which he replied, 'No, the girl did a good job.' I still don't know if that was a promotion or demotion from the boy.

CRITICAL REFLECTION QUESTION
What do you observe about the life of a trainee cardiothoracic surgeon in this case study?

It had been a particularly busy week at work and I was absolutely exhausted. I had been coming in early most days and leaving late—my husband and I had been married six months but we were like ships passing in the night at times. And he was always incredulous as to why I gave so much to surgery. I had to if I wanted to keep my position and stay in the boss's good graces. But I also wanted to, well, because I loved my job. I always enjoyed the hospital early in the morning; it was quiet enough to let me catch up with work that needed doing, going through CT scan results or examining the angiograms for that day's operations. And it was rather quaint: I always felt like there was some excitement in the air for the day. Like a promise of a brand-new opportunity for us all to do amazing things.

My phone rang and the hospital number flashed up. 'Hello, doctor, switchboard here, just putting you through to the ED consultant.' It was just after 6.30 a.m.; the ED consultant usually only started at 8 a.m., which meant some disaster was taking place they had rushed in for. Strange how the minutiae of the way the hospital works becomes so second nature to you that any deviation gives you all the information you need to know about what is to follow.

I was right to be suspicious. There was a full cardiac arrest happening in ED. A man had fallen asleep outside at a friend's house after a few beers on what happened to be the coldest night of the year and the winter solstice. He was found just before 6 a.m. by the newspaper delivery man in the driveway of the house and an ambulance had scooped him up and brought him to our hospital.

When your body temperature drops, your heartbeat first slows and then degenerates into something called ventricular fibrillation. Rather than beating regularly, the heart twitches or shakes (fibrillates), which means that it cannot pump blood forwards. When I entered the ED, I saw the team pushing life into his cold body, his temperature barely reading 30 degrees Celsius (normal body temperature is a balmy 37 degrees). The ED consultant relayed the story to me but before he finished, I asked him what I assumed he'd called me here to do: 'You want ECMO?' I have a habit of leaping ahead in conversations, my brain making the connections faster than it can tell my mouth to wait, a habit that other people find frustrating at best or rude at worst.

ECMO is extracorporeal membrane oxygenation or a form of long-term heart–lung machine support. We can use it for dozens of things, like a failing heart or lungs, but one of the most daring indications for it is when CPR isn't working. This is serious last-ditch-attempt medicine, undies-on-the-outside heroics. I looked at the guy for a minute while a nurse was giving chest compressions. He was young and he was cold. The cold had probably preserved his organs when his heart stopped, so his brain should be safe. He was only 25 years old; it was a daring race for ECMO or death. I chose ECMO.

I rang my boss on call and told him the story as I hurriedly directed people to get this man up to theatre. I spat out the story at a million miles an hour down the phone and told him, 'I'm going to put him on ECMO; everyone is getting ready now,' feeling like I had already made the decision as if I were the one in charge, not just the registrar.

'Crack on then,' the boss told me as I entered the lift to get up to theatre.

As the doors to theatre opened, it was crammed full of everyone who could possibly help. I loved the sight of an all-hands-on-deck situation like this. The CPR continued as we transferred the man's cold, lifeless body to centre stage in the operating theatre. Packages of instruments and pipes were being opened expeditiously and I rushed to scrub up, ready to push life back into his body.

ECMO is usually put in peripherally, meaning we access the blood vessels of the groin or the neck to pass pipes around two and a half centimetres in diameter to take blood away from the body via an artery, warm it, clean it and oxygenate it and then return it by another pipe in a vein. I knew I could put ECMO in quickly via the femoral artery and vein of the groin so I splashed antiseptic on his right groin and covered it with the blue drapes. His whole body bounced up and down while the rest of the team continued the CPR, keeping him alive, and as I put my hands on the landmarks to show myself where the vessels were, I was taken aback at just how cold he was.

I plunged a needle into the groin, getting a tiny flash of blood that let me know I was in the vessel. But as I tried to pass a wire that would act as a guide for the pipe to travel along, I kept meeting resistance. I tried again, and again the same thing. I took a breath and tried one last time but to no avail. 'Fuck it!' I said in exasperation. 'I think he's too cold, the vessels are all shut down.' At the same time, my boss came into the room and we stared at the patient, and the monitor for a second. 'I can open his chest?' I ventured and the boss yelled back at me, 'Okay, do that!' as he went to wash his hands and help.

A tonne more instruments were opened and I threw more antiseptic on the chest as the CPR was halted after what had seemed like hours. I thrust the scalpel into the skin and down onto the sternum. The nurse handed me the saw and as I buzzed it once to test it it screeched over the top of the noise in theatre. The sternum split apart as the saw screamed through it; the scrub nurse swapped the saw for a pair of scissors into my boss's hands; thankfully, he was now standing opposite me on the left side. We took it in turns squeezing the heart, providing internal compressions to try to keep this guy alive while we worked.

I quickly put a purse string in the aorta and the right atrium and thrust the bypass cannulae into the heart. We connected the pipes to the machine and yelled over the top of everyone in theatre to the perfusionist, 'Go on!', meaning to go on to ECMO, and with that, blood flowed out of him and into the machine, returning just as quickly, restoring a kind of life.

For the first time that morning, I felt like I could breathe as I took in what had happened. My boss and I looked at each other and started to tally up just how lucky this guy was. He had fallen asleep on the coldest night of the year, had been found on a paper route, had gotten to hospital when a senior ED doctor was present and when I was already in the hospital and other essential staff had just begun to arrive so that we could put him on ECMO and save his life.

And with that, we both burst out laughing.

'Holy shit, this is the luckiest guy on the planet!'

Luck doesn't seem like something that should have a place in an operating theatre. But in reality, it sure as hell factors in more than we would like. Sometimes, in the face of all adversity, things go better than you could ever imagine they could. And sometimes, for reasons that will never be known, things go unbelievably badly.

I was starting to hit my stride, doing more and more operating myself and feeling more and more confident, like I was finally getting the hang of this heart surgery business. Like I may finally, one day, be a fully fledged consultant cardio-thoracic surgeon. And damn it felt good. But that is the thing about heart surgery. Just when you think everything's going well, heart surgery likes to remind you that it can all change in an instant.

CASE 7

I was about to do my first aortic valve replacement myself from start to finish. I was very aware of the enormity of this, having spent a couple of years as the trainee, slowly being allowed to do more and more. What starts as some suturing here and there eventually turns into three or four hours of an entire operation—every incision, every stitch. These increments are, of course, predominantly about building skill but it's also about building confidence and I was sure I had both.

Gladys was in hospital, awaiting her surgery. Her aortic valve had been slowly fusing shut for many years, a condition called aortic stenosis. It makes it difficult for the heart to pump against the stiff and narrowed valve. Eventually, it can't cope and the heart starts to struggle, leaving people with aortic stenosis straining to do things they used to do or with pain in the chest for even the more mundane things in life, like climbing a flight of stairs. She was waiting for surgery at home, hoping the hospital would call and say that her day had arrived, but as so often happens, a month turned into two and then stretched out to nearly six months.

A surgery that was supposed to be urgent was downgraded as the perpetually overwhelmed public health system struggled to keep up.

She couldn't wait any longer and came to hospital, struggling to breathe and tired of waiting. We made the decision to keep her in hospital until her surgery could be done, knowing that not only was she too sick to wait, it was the best way to make sure she wasn't waiting any longer than necessary.

I saw her the night before her surgery. She could have been my own grandmother, tucked up in a hospital bed, telling me stories about her family. The last thing she wanted to talk about was her heart surgery, even to the point that, when I wanted to tell her about the possible risks of the surgery, she put her hand up and said to me, 'If I die, I die. All I know is that I can't live like this anymore.'

I got ready for the surgery, and with my mask and loupes (custom-made glasses that magnify everything I see two and a half times) in place, I pulled the operating headlight on to my head and tightened it. It was like a crown, with the wearer designated as the surgeon in charge for the case. As I stood at the sink washing my hands for the five minutes it takes to scrub, I went through the steps of the surgery in my head. Sternotomy, pericardium, give the heparin, cannulate, cross-clamp, aortotomy and so on. This was a habit that would follow me for years, like a sports star imagining a successful manoeuvre in their mind.

And that was exactly how the surgery went, each step following after the other. My boss, opposite me as my assistant, offered helpful hints here and there, making sure that I was on track at every turn. He was my teacher, my cheerleader and my safety net. And, although I try never to think this because I don't want to jinx myself, the surgery was going well. Really well, in fact.

The valve was in and it was time to take the cross-clamp off and let blood back into the heart so it could resume doing the job it was meant to do. It's the most beautiful part of heart surgery: the large clamp that sits across the aorta, effectively isolating the heart from the rest of the circulation, keeping the heart bloodless for the surgery, eases off and blood rushes back into the heart. To watch a heart spring to life is my absolute favourite sight in the world, partly because of the magnificence of physiology at work but also because, if you've done the operation well, the heart will just work. There's no greater endorsement than that.

On this my first aortic valve replacement, I eased the cross-clamp off, telling the perfusionist that the heart was now freed, in a sense. Just as I had hoped, although the ventricles wobbled a bit for a few beats as the heart tried to find its rhythm again, it quickly started to beat in the perfectly choreographed cadence it was meant to.

My relief was short-lived. While I breathed a sigh of relief that the heart worked, my attention was about to be diverted to something else: alongside the aorta, blood was welling up at a much faster rate than it should. I could feel my own heart start to race as my boss and I tried to work out what the hell was going on. When something like this happens in theatre, the mood change is palpable for everyone.

'Swap sides,' my boss said, an indication that he thought something was wrong enough that he needed to be in the driver's seat and not me. I could feel the heat of terror rising up under my gown. On the assistant's side of the table now, I watched as my boss looked for the problem. The only way to get a good look at it was to stop the heart once more, to give us a bloodless field. And so, not long after it had been liberated, the heart was again cross-clamped while we tried to work out what the problem was and, more importantly, fix it.

It was hard to push the thought out of my head that I had done something wrong. While focusing on what was going on in the moment, I was also simultaneously replaying everything. Was my suturing not good enough? Did I cut something I shouldn't have? I tried to reassure myself that everything had been done under the watchful eye of my consultant, checking every step of the way. And more importantly, I tried to convince myself that, whatever the problem was, we could fix it.

With the heart quiet and bloodless, the problem soon became evident. One of the most feared complications in cardiac surgery had happened—a tear had started inside the heart, plunging down deep inside it, disrupting the heart so that it simply could not work anymore. The heat of terror quickly turned into ice-cold dread, knowing that this was a complication that was hard to come back from.

For the next three hours, we tried everything to put her heart back together. Holding myself together so that all of the emotions I had wouldn't spill out was as hard as holding her heart together. Nothing worked, and my first aortic valve replacement became my first on-table death.

My boss sat down next to me. He turned me around in my swivel chair and inched close to me, his legs awkwardly either side of mine and took my hand in his. While I kept my head bowed, so that he couldn't see my discomfort, he reassured me that we had done everything we could. 'I would have told you if you were fucking it up. Some days, you can do everything right and still have this happen.' He was right: this is the way high-stakes surgeries like this can unfold. The hard thing for us all to accept is that some days, no matter how well you do your job, in surgery bad things can still happen. Despite that, the painful guilt when someone doesn't make it is a burden that is, quite frankly, overwhelming.

'Welcome to heart surgery, kid.'

CRITICAL REFLECTION QUESTION

What do you observe about the life of a trainee cardiothoracic surgeon in this case study?

When I was a really junior doctor, saving someone's life was kind of a nebulous concept. You looked after patients but you weren't really that person who does the high-stakes, truly lifesaving things that make you feel able to walk out of the hospital at the end of the day knowing that you saved someone. What was also a far-off, hazy concept to grasp was that you could also be responsible for not making the save, or even directly contributing to someone's ill health or worse. It is a cliché, but the saying 'With great power comes great responsibility' seems a more than apt way to describe being a surgeon. It seemed particularly relevant while learning to be a surgeon.

As I learnt more and got more and more skills under my belt, I started to feel like a real doctor, a real surgeon. It wasn't arrogance; it was more a feeling of pride and accomplishment as well as a kind of safety, knowing that if someone was sick, if they were hurt and needed me, I actually had half a chance of truly being able to help them. The hypothermic man whose heart had stopped—had I met him even just a year earlier, I don't know if I would have been able to help him. A year before, he may not have walked out of hospital, a wound down the centre of his chest the only sign that something bad had happened to him one cold night.

It started to dawn on me what an immense privilege it was to be let into someone's life like that. In surgery, you are privy to some of the most intimate moments of people's existence. You see the fear in their eyes as they face open-heart surgery or, worse, when they're told there is nothing you can do. On the other hand, you are there for the sheer elation and glee when you get to tell someone's loved ones that their son or daughter has made it, especially when it's against all odds.

As you go from strength to strength in your career, you start to shift from being a passive observer in these moments to an instrument of their outcome. The more you learn the more you can do, the greater the ability you have to directly impact on what happens to someone. All of a sudden, you start to realise that you can actually save a life.

On ward rounds, I began to feel this immense sense of pride as I saw patients on whom I had actually done their surgery. I felt like I was truly their surgeon, not just some kid who helped a little bit by holding a retractor here and there or charting the medications they needed. Not that those things aren't important. But I was just so pleased that I was actually able to make a difference to someone's life. It was the greatest reward ever.

When I was among other trainees, we'd regale one another with stories of the amazing saves we'd had or the impressively complicated surgeries we'd performed. In true surgeon style, the conversations weren't exactly light-hearted and congratu-latory. They were competitive and full of one-upmanship; we learnt early on that being hyper-competitive was most defi-nitely part of being a heart surgeon. But while everyone shared their wins with wild abandon, nobody ever talked about how hard it was. Nobody ever talked about the moments of doubt. And not once did I ever hear someone say their actions hurt someone, or even worse.

Did we stay quiet on our missteps to save face or were we too afraid to admit to fragility even amid our burgeoning skills as surgeons, that not everything always went to plan? Therein was the great responsibility of what we were doing. While we were slogging it out, working all day, studying and practising all night to be better surgeons, the more chances to use our craft and our skills meant more chances to hurt someone.

Many studies have repeatedly shown that when surgical trainees are supervised in the operating theatre, their inexperience does not place the patient at increased risk. Cardiac surgery, though, is unique among many other types of surgery in that there is a genuine risk of someone dying on your operating table. Roughly one in a hundred people will die having heart surgery, the risk increasing with the more risky surgeries. And no matter how good you are, no matter how experienced or careful, sometimes things go wrong for reasons that are unclear.

That first death on my operating table wasn't a wake-up call; I went into heart surgery with my eyes wide open as to what was at stake. I knew I needed to make sure that everything I did was perfect to minimise the risk of bad things happening. The hard thing was that this risk would never be zero.

There is a saying that every surgeon carries within themselves a tiny cemetery, filled with reminders of the patients they have lost. Over the course of a career, that is quite a burden to bear, particularly if, like me, you were going to be performing some of the most high-risk surgeries possible.

My first big save and my first big loss on the operating table happened in such close proximity to each other, as if to show me how high the highs could be and how desperately devastating the lows. I have immense pride in the wins, and an incredible sense of accomplishment for not just what I was achieving but for being part of a remarkable team. But the lows, those losses, I think, were probably there to teach me so much more. I think those times were there to remind me never, ever to take my eyes off the prize.

5

TRAINEE REGISTRAR
Clinically dead

Surgery always seems like you have someone's life in your hands. But very often, it feels like surgery had my life in its hands. Everything was centred around surgery; everything came second to surgery. Every day, every minute, of my world was determined by what my career needed. Including being in the hands of the training board of cardiothoracic surgery, what felt like a group of faceless men who would sit around and decide what was next for you, for your life and for your career.

In order to get the most out of training, every two years we had to move to a different hospital. The idea was that you were exposed to different methods, different surgeons or even different problems. If you were from Sydney or Melbourne, it might mean moving to a hospital just down the road. But if, like me, you were from Perth, it almost inevitably meant moving across the country or even to New Zealand. There was an illusion of choice—you could ask for where you wanted to go but the reality was that you were told where to go and the rest of your life had to fall into line.

I arrived to the big-city life in Sydney in the height of summer, checking into a hotel on the edge of Kings Cross, the infamous night-life district while I looked for a house. I had left my husband back in Perth while he finished his training. I wasn't that familiar with Sydney, aside from knowing the tourist hotspots of Bondi Beach and the Opera House. I didn't realise it initially, but the entrance to my hotel backed on to a brothel and a nightclub's rear exit. The streets outside bustled with revellers and police sirens from dusk until dawn. It was a big change from the laid-back 'burbs I was used to.

I didn't know anyone in Sydney, no friends and no family. I'd only visited the city maybe twice in my life and now I was navigating starting a new job and hunting for a new house while simultaneously being perpetually available for the heavy workload at one of the busiest and most prestigious cardiothoracic units in the country. Trying to steer myself through the cutthroat (and painfully expensive) Sydney real estate market while at the same time fielding calls from the hospital was trying, to say the least.

There was no easing into any of this; that's not how medicine works. Whether or not it should be like this is a different question, it was just the way it had to be. You have to hit the ground running on the very first day, personally and professionally. No house? Too bad, you don't need one when you'll basically be living at the hospital. Not sure where your ward is? Work it out. Got locked in a stairwell because you didn't know which floor to get out? Tough. Starting a new job meant begging for a locker in theatre change-rooms and figuring out how to get swipe cards so I could actually access theatre and wards to do my work. I tried my hardest not to be overwhelmed and just focus on what I was there to do, but I couldn't help feeling alone, confused and longing for the familiarity of home.

I was in the thick of things from the beginning, on call on my very first day. There was no 'Let's just get you settled' lag time here. My phone rang at 10 p.m. on my first day to tell me I'd be flying to a country town a couple of hours away to perform emergency surgery. From the second I set foot in that hospital, I was to be available all the time. Even if I wasn't on call, being part of a busy cardiothoracic unit meant that it was always all hands on deck. We simply needed everyone to be there in order to get the work done.

A feeling of being overwhelmed started to grow each and every day. I was drowning in the rush to find a house, to make friends, to find my way around the hospital and, most of all, to prove myself to my new consultants. Instead of feeling like I was rising to the occasion, I felt like I was just a great big fuck-up. I couldn't find a house, I was filled with anxiety that I wasn't good enough professionally, and I was in a constant state of exhaustion, from working up to one hundred hours a week. Who was I? I knew I was good at my job, but here I couldn't shake the feeling that I simply wasn't myself.

To be in a unit that is a world leader in the field was supposed to be my dream come true. I was thrilled to be there. But as the days rolled by and I felt less and less like I belonged there—personally and professionally—I almost started to forget why I loved my work so much in the first place. The stress of everything—being alone, feeling inadequate, finding my feet in a new and unimaginably busy place—seemed to dull some of my love for what I thought I wanted to do.

CASE 8

One stormy Saturday night, it was transplant time and we took off from Sydney to fly three hours north to pick up a heart and lungs from a donor who had died and whose family had made the courageous decision to save someone else's life. I used to call this plane the 'stretcher plane'; it was a small, twin-jet plane that was used for medical retrievals, so it had an old stretcher down one side of the cabin. It may have technically originally been a private jet but there was no luxury in sight. I hated that plane; it was relatively old and uncomfortable, and I spent many hours in it, flying all around the country.

As the stretcher plane took off, the stormy weather threw us around. My heart was racing and my breathing was heavy and, although I didn't realise it at the time, every bump was matched by me with an 'eep' or an 'oh' as I let the fear squeak out. The transplant nurse on the flight would many months later tell me how she listened to my every little gasp and laughed, wondering what the hell I was doing in this job if I hated flying for retrievals so much.

It was actually a fair question. The flights in these tiny planes were always anxiety-inducing for me, as someone who is not a fan of tiny planes. But as soon as we would touch down, the anxiety would be gone and I would be a different person, back in charge.

After we landed on this stormy day and our equipment had been safely unloaded, a taxi took us to the hospital. In the back of the taxi at 3 a.m., I was in control as I did a final review of the medical notes of the donor. I looked through everything with great detail—how they had died, what medicines they were currently receiving, what their blood group was and who the recipient was going to be. The scared little girl in the stretcher plane was replaced by a confident heart surgeon.

To be an organ donor, you have to die in a very specific set of circumstances. For starters, it has to be in an intensive care unit. The ICU is a highly sub-specialised area of the hospital where, as the name suggests, patients receive intensive care, such as being ventilated when they can't breathe for themselves. Virtually every organ system in the body can receive the highest level of support by the expert doctors and nurses in an ICU.

But the one organ system that is so elusive that we can't replace it as we can most other organs is the brain. When the brain is so severely damaged to the point where its loss of function is completely irreversible, we call this 'brain death'. When the brain is dead, that person is legally declared deceased. Even when the brain is 'dead', the heart, the lungs and the other vital organs can continue to function for some days after, reflexively. This means that after brain death, if that person has healthy organs otherwise, they can be an organ donor.

In Australia, we have an opt-in system where nobody is presumed to be a donor. After someone is declared brain dead, independent organ donation specialists will ask the family for permission for the deceased to be an organ donor. Sometimes for one or two organs, sometimes for many or all of the organs that can be donated. It is a highly regulated system to make sure that everything is done ethically and that the care of the person who may become a donor always takes priority. It is one of the most heartbreaking yet simultaneously uplifting things that can happen in a hospital.

We arrived at the donor hospital: me, my assistant who was a more junior registrar and one of the transplant nurses. In the operating theatre, the donor had already arrived, as had the abdominal surgical team. Two different surgical teams attend when the liver and the kidneys are also being donated; we all stay in our area of specialty.

Before we started, everyone gathered around as the coordinator prepared to brief us. This was where we would once again hear all the details as to how this patient had wound up here. They were never good stories, compounded by the fact that the donors were often relatively young. There were accidents and fistfights, sudden ruptures of aneurysms in the brain that had been ticking time bombs, or other unusual medical conditions. In those briefings, some of the most poignant stories left even battle-hardened surgeons misty-eyed. We're always there to do a job but we never forget that this is the ultimate gift someone will receive off the back of another family's ultimate loss.

Even though this person is legally deceased, they are treated exactly like we would treat any other person: with great care and dignity. There is no haphazard anything; it is still a surgical operation like any other, just that this time the outcome is going to be very different. The patient is 'prepped and draped'—where we paint their chest and abdomen with antiseptic solution and then carefully place surgical drapes over their body so that the precious organs inside are protected from the bacteria and other insults of the outside world. The draping is important to me, psychologically. Not just there to create a sterile field, the drapes are a thin but important barrier between the harrowing stories and emotionally charged events and my need to do a job. With the patient's face covered, I can, for just a moment, focus on the job I am there to do and not focus on the sadness that has probably devastated another family.

By this stage I was well into my first year in Sydney, and my abdominal surgery colleague and I had spent many nights together at operating tables around the country doing this exact operation. While we both venture inside the body, I into the chest and he into the abdomen, the conversation is light and jovial in stark contrast to the seriousness of what we're doing. Doctors and nurses are known for this distancing and, as cold as it may seem, it keeps us safe from the burden of others' misery and allows us to focus on the very important task at hand.

I sawed open the sternum, just like I would in any heart surgery, and exposed the heart, beating away in the pericardium, by cutting the fibrous sac straight down the middle. As expected, the heart was beautiful; it works so perfectly. I checked everything about it—how well it was pumping, looking for plaque in the arteries and feeling for undiscovered problems that might make the heart too sick for transplant into someone else. The lungs sat separately to the heart in their own kind of sacs, the pleura. They got opened too and I felt every centimetre of the lungs and marvelled at their beautiful pink hue, untouched by city living or cigarette smoke. It was all good news, so I unscrubbed to call my boss and tell him that the organs were perfect and that we should be back in just under four hours.

In an organ retrieval, the abdominal team goes first initially, dividing the attachments for the liver and kidneys inside the belly in preparation for their eventual removal. My abdominal colleague was speedy, and I barely had time for a toilet break and to hunt through the hospital tearoom for some kind of food like stale biscuits or two-day-old bread. Once the abdominal team was ready for me to do the final steps before the climactic part of this surgery, it was my turn to begin the process of liberating the heart and lungs.

I love this operation, not just because of what it represents but also because, to do it, you have to have an intimate understanding of the anatomy of the heart and lungs. Each part needs to be separated from the surrounding structures where there's just the tiniest of spaces between them, meaning that the margin for error is even smaller. With the heart and lungs partially freed from their body, the final step is to place small tubes into the heart. One goes into the aorta and delivers a medicine called cardioplegia and the other into the pulmonary artery, delivering pneumoplegia. Each solution contains medicines and other substances to preserve the organs, trying to suspend them in time and make them safe for their journey to someone else. The abdominal surgeon makes similar arrangements for the liver and kidneys. And then, all of a sudden, we're ready for the final part of this surgery.

I always shout out for quiet here because this is the most frantic and critical part of the surgery and the theatre is always noisy with chatter. There are three steps I have to do here: stop blood coming back to the heart by tying off the vena cava; clamp the aorta with a long, silver clamp; and cut the heart on the left atrium to stop blood blowing the heart up like a balloon and causing damage. After that, the drugs need to get into the heart and lungs, preserving them as perfectly as we can. Any missteps in these moments may damage these beautiful organs to a point where they may not be able to be used.

But that day, everything went smoothly. The donor coordinator yelled out above the business of the theatre, 'Cross-clamp time, 0415'. A clock had just started: the heart had four hours to be implanted in the recipient and reconnected to blood supply, the lungs six hours. Going longer than this increases the chances that the new organs in their new body will struggle to work. From the second I place that cross-clamp on, the organs are dying and nothing can interrupt the process.

The medicines take several minutes to complete their work, and the second they were finished I started removing the organs from the chest. No other surgery makes me quiet; normally I chat away while I operate but not that day. There is no room for making a mistake; a wrong cut can be devastating and irreparable. It took me about ten minutes to have everything free and then I was holding the heart and lungs in my arms.

To get them home, each organ is placed in a bag, which is placed in another bag and into yet another bag. Every organ has three bags to ensure they will be safe and remain sterile. Once safely in their bags, the organs are buried under ice in an esky, the standard kind of esky you'd normally fill with beer and barbecue foods. On weekend nights when I'd walk in or out of the hospital with an esky or two, invariably someone whose party had wound up at the ED would ask for a beer. Having carried such precious cargo in them has changed the way I look at eskys forever.

The storms had subsided by this stage, so I didn't need to give a repeat performance of anxiety on the flight home.

Not outwardly, anyway. At the airport, we were met by police cars that took us back to the hospital with lights and sirens. Strangely enough, being in a police car careening down the motorway is not nearly as anxiety-inducing for me as being on a plane. We screamed into the hospital and raced from the elevator to the operating theatre where two people were getting a new chance at life, the surgery already begun. And I got some good news.

'Nikki, we've accepted another donor offer. You need to head out again at 8 a.m., so have some food and do a quick ward round before you go.'

My watch told me the bad news: it was 6:50 a.m. and sleep was a distant memory from two days ago. I was the kind of tired that you not only felt in your bones, but in your soul. And it felt like shit.

CRITICAL REFLECTION QUESTION
What do you observe about the life of a trainee cardiothoracic surgeon in this case study?

'Please be empty, please be empty, please be empty.'

I knew that any second my tears were about to escape, and I just needed to make it to a (I hoped) empty theatre change-room before that happened. Because you never cry at work. You can cry in your car in a pinch or when you get home, but never at work where your vulnerability and brokenness can be seen by everyone. If they see that you're weak, then at best you're a fun toy for them to torture and at worst you're unworthy of your job.

My consultant had just finished destroying me in a packed operating theatre. Again. He had made a bit of a habit of making sure the entire room of ten or so people knew that he didn't think much of me.

'You fucking useless bitch,' he spewed at me. Many years down the track, I still don't understand why. I had made a split-second decision to operate on one of his patients who was bleeding far too much after open-heart surgery. It turned out to be the right call, but it wasn't what he had wanted me to do. I would have had to have followed his order except that at that moment of making the call to him, I couldn't get hold of him. Regardless of the appropriateness of what I had done, he had a difference of opinion. Which is not to say that I was correct and he was wrong; there are often different ways to reach the same outcome.

Nevertheless, I will never forget my back against the computer, the keyboard digging into me and me wishing that I could disappear through the wall as this man yelled at me in front of a captive audience as the patient was being taken back to the intensive care unit. I could hear their gasps and see the shock on the faces of my colleagues as he erupted. At one point, in his rage, he even managed to throw in a dig at how difficult life must have been for my then-husband, dealing with my insubordination.

I had been around long enough to know to say nothing

in these situations. There was nothing I was going to be able to say in the midst of that tirade to diffuse the situation. I knew enough angry people in my life to know at least this much: the damage would be attenuated if I just stayed quiet and focused on the feeling of the keyboard in my back than on the sting of the very public lashing I was receiving. And eventually it did stop when I suppose he tired of the vitriol and just walked out of the operating theatre, leaving the air sullied with the bile of his outburst.

One of my colleagues who was witness to the whole event, whom I had known since I was a teenager, tried to put an arm around me and said, 'You did not deserve that'. And it was that kindness that broke me. Not the anger, not the barbs and insults. For some reason, the thing that made me run out of the theatre as quickly as I could to get to where my tears wouldn't be seen was the humanity of an old friend.

Since that day seemed to not want to cut me any slack, just as the tears started to tumble out of my eyes the change-room door flung open to a group of student nurses, who looked shocked and terrified to see my raw, ugly distress. All I wanted was an empty room so nobody had to witness my breakdown. I heard one of them call out to me as I raced to a toilet stall that I could lock prying eyes out of. And then I broke the 'Don't cry at work' rule and let all the hurt go.

Truth be told, it wasn't just that one day, that one hu-miliation. Those tears were all of the darkness that I had been carrying around for months. The loneliness and isolation.

The working hours so long I could barely remember the last meal that wasn't from a vending machine. The sickness and suffering of others that my job required me to marinate in. The sacrifice that was inevitable for a surgical career. It was all gushing out now uncontrollably, and there was no way I could pack it back inside me. The darkness was finally roaming free.

The only good fortune that day brought me was I didn't have to work that night, a rare but desperately needed reprieve. Those tears followed me home, and I lay in the shower for what seemed like the whole night, crying alone, trying to dull the pain and the emotions with a bottle of shitty white wine.

The next morning, my eyes were puffy from the tears and fatigue of not just the day before but of everything. When the alarm pierced my wine- and exhaustion-induced sleep, I threw my phone across the bedroom and screamed at it to shut the fuck up. I couldn't get up. I just couldn't touch my feet to the floor; it was as if it was on fire and I just wanted to stay in the safety of my bed. It was fear that gripped me, that prevented me from facing yet another day that could leave me broken in the locked toilet stall of a theatre change-room.

I did the only thing I knew I could muster the energy and forward momentum to do. I called in sick to work.

In medicine, there is a joke that if you call in sick to work, you had better provide a death certificate since the only legitimate reason for not turning up is that you are deceased. It might get a few giggles when you say it, but the reality is there is nothing at all amusing about that maxim. I *felt* dead that day: numb, and immobilised by fear, exhaustion and a sadness so big that it had engulfed me. I was entitled to and desperately in need of that day off. It didn't stop the immense guilt that came from saying I wouldn't be in, leaving my colleagues to pull up the slack that my absence would leave, despite the fact I was so broken I wouldn't be any use anyway. I also couldn't shake the feeling that everyone would know the reason I wasn't there was that I had been freshly flayed by my boss and I was 'breakable', making me utterly hopeless as a heart surgeon by default.

I still don't know how I managed to see through the fog that day and ask for help but I did. I rang my GP to slot into an afternoon appointment that day. During that appointment the surgeon in me protested things 'weren't really that bad' and I was probably 'overreacting'. The doctor stared at me just long enough to coax the tears out once more and, along with their liberation, I blurted out everything that was wrong with my life, which led us both to the same inevitable conclusion. I was not coping. I was not fine. I was not overreacting.

I was not okay.

Even now, after so much time has passed, just telling this story makes me question if it really was that bad and if I was just as weak as they thought I was. The degree of gaslighting in my profession to ensure we carry on no matter how wounded we are is hard to overstate.

***

I always was and always will be immensely proud to be a doctor. I feel that there are very few other jobs in the world that let you take care of other people the way those of us who work in health care do. That need to care for another human, sometimes during their most harrowing hour, is at the heart of everything we do. Whether it be the surgeon who performs the operation, the clerk who ensures your medical records are properly maintained, the nurse who takes your blood pressure or the person who brings you your meals, it's because we desperately want you to be looked after. That is, by and large, why we're there to begin with.

One of my favourite nurses, one of the nicest people I ever had the pleasure of working with, had the biggest heart of anyone I've met. She and I would sit in her office during quiet times, gossiping about the royal family, making plans to streamline patients' journeys through our ward and sharing photos of our lives outside the hospital. Before she was in charge of my ward, she was an ICU nurse, looking after the sickest and most vulnerable people in a hospital at any given time. ICU nurses are highly trained; they supervise the life-support systems that keep a patient suspended in life. It's a highly technical and academic branch of nursing and some of the finest nurses I've worked with come from the ICU.

But amid the constant drone of machines that ping and alarm, of whirring pumps and crisp white linen that define the ICU, my favourite nurse always found the humanity to care for her patients. In one of our afternoon chats, she told me how she became an expert groomer when looking after her patients in ICU. She'd ask the patients' families how they liked their hair, if they waxed or shaved their legs, and then turned her room into a kind of beauty salon. In between administering drugs to support the heart or induce unconsciousness to heal the ailing body, she would style hair, pluck eyebrows and shave legs. 'It was the least I could do,' she told me. 'After all, they're fighting for their fucking lives; I just wanted them to look like their usual selves.' I told her that if I was ever in ICU how I like my hair done and not to pluck my eyebrows too thin. She promised not to shave them off as a joke.

The strange thing about medicine is that, when it comes to kindness, we can deliver it in spades to our patients but to one another? That's an impossible ask. Let me be clear: this isn't just isolated to doctors. Every profession and department in the hospital loves to pick on its own and on each other. We push each other to breaking point, until someone is crying in the change-rooms or even worse. We are all too often completely and utterly devoid of empathy towards one another and, when you're a trainee, you're on the receiving end more than most.

***

Somehow, I returned to work after feeling like I was dead inside. Truth be told, I was just trying to survive every day. The workload and the culture of humiliation and belittlement were making it hard. Most days, I felt a little like I was going through the motions. Each time the phone rang and it was work, I could literally feel my body tense up in preparation for either exhaustion or evisceration. I think I was living in a perpetual state of fear.

I was in the emergency department at around 4 a.m. one morning, waiting for a patient who had been in a car accident and sustained severe chest injuries. Although the lights were dimmed in the department to simulate night time, it was no less alive and awake for patients and staff alike. I sat on the chair on the flight deck, a raised platform where doctors and nurses field phone calls, write notes and, in my case, sit and wait for a patient to arrive while raiding lollies in a kidney dish on the desk to keep me awake.

I could hear a bit of a commotion between two doctors next to the flight deck. I eavesdropped on the conversation as it got increasingly tense. One of the RMOs had just seen someone with a minor hand injury. The poor patient had driven a nail through his own fingernail and, thanks to a busy ED, he'd only just been seen, many hours later. The injury sounded very unimpressive by medical standards although it's safe to say the patient probably didn't think so.

Years before, I had been a plastic surgery registrar on one of my many registrar rotations through surgical specialties. In fact, I toyed with that career pathway to hand surgery. Hand injuries, major and minor, make up a large part of your on-call burden. Injuries like this, to the nail and the nail bed, often needed a short operation to fix any cuts in the nail bed, so that as the nail grows over the injury it does so straight and normally. It was about as far from an emergency as you can get in plastic surgery.

This was the view shared by the resident, who I knew had been the plastic surgery RMO recently. She knew not only that the injury was not critical but also that the plastic surgery registrar on-call is one of the busiest jobs in the hospital and those registrars put in some of the longest hours of anyone. In short, they are flogged within an inch of their lives. To that end, she had suggested to her registrar that they keep the patient in the ED for the morning plastics ward round just a few short hours away and let the plastics registrar get some rest. A plan I silently supported wholeheartedly, having been that dead-tired person not so long ago and having waved at the plastics registrar going home and looking ghastly as I walked into the hospital half an hour earlier. The poor bastard needed more than a few hours' sleep; he needed a few weeks.

The ED registrar crossed her arms and smirked. 'He's paid to be on call. Which means he's paid to be awake. If we're up, he's up.' She proceeded to continue to demand that the RMO refer the patient for review and demand the plastics registrar's attendance in the department. The RMO told her it was wrong, and a stand-off ensued until the registrar said, 'Fine, I'll call him myself and you can explain to the consultant tomorrow why you won't make referrals to in-patient specialties'.

What a bitch, I thought to myself. If the tables had been turned and we were waking her up when she had been on-call all night, she would have been rightly infuriated. While ED doctors work incredibly hard, they predominantly do shift work; surgical registrars stay up all night and then operate all day. Sleep is for the dead, we're often told. My trauma patient arrived just as I was trying not to vocalise how cruel I thought the registrar was being, despite it technically being none of my business. Which is probably a good thing because, had I said something, I would have gotten a serve from her at best and a formal complaint at worst, because if we can't upset you face to face, hospital staff will make a complaint and let the bureaucracy of a flawed complaints management system finish you off.

Where was the compassion? That same registrar joined me on my trauma case where she not only was the patient's doctor, she was a soothing voice in his ear, reassuring him that we would take care of him and that everything would be fine. She offered to call his wife and asked repeatedly if he had any pain because if he did, she could fix it. Not that long ago, she had been deliberately inflicting psychological pain on a colleague. What a strange juxtaposition.

Do we have a finite capacity for compassion that we prioritise for our patients over our colleagues? I think it's entirely possible. I know that in moments of stress, tiredness or frustration, my phone voice has degenerated from professional to overtly irritated. Even the nicest and most patient doctors have done this. But the conversation I had overheard was something different altogether: it was almost sadistic.

And that callousness is not isolated to that conversation, or that person. On the receiving end, or watching other registrars be publicly or privately lynched, sometimes you see a little moment of glee when the aggressor strikes. It's why you never, ever cry at work in case the person yelling at you is hoping for that pleasure of seeing you crack. It's why that day I ran to the change-rooms for shelter.

Although these moments aren't common, they aren't rare either. And I don't think they come from the cold, dark hearts of people who like inflicting pain on their colleagues. I think they come from a system and a culture that, generation after generation, breaks any spirit of kindness we have. It makes us a number, a position, a cog in a machine that doesn't really care whether you thrive or just survive, so long as the roster spot is filled and the work gets done. Even the kindest soul can turn into someone who demands an exhausted colleague attend at 4 a.m. unnecessarily because we have been shattered by a system that is so broken and unforgiving itself.

* * *

A colleague, a fellow surgical registrar in another specialty, once asked me point blank whether, if I had my time over again, I would still do heart surgery. And on the day he asked, I looked at him, put on my most convincing smile and threw my hands up in the air, shouting, 'Of course I would! I love it!'

I lied. Every cell in my body was calling me a liar for not saying how much regret I had. Granted, on the day that he asked me, I was having a bad day. In fact, I was having a bad year. I felt like I had finally been ground down by all of the bad things that had happened, all of the sadness I had seen and all of the frustrations lumped on me by the system.

I'm not alone. In fact, I'm fairly certain the reason my colleague had asked me is that he too had this pit of regret. Some days that pit was massive and some days it was just a little puddle of all the things that you've hated over the years: the weddings and funerals you've missed, the broken relationships, the death, the burden of responsibility, the bureaucracy.

Eventually, I reached my own breaking point for the first time in my career, and had support groups for surgeons, or even just someone not entrenched in the system, been around at that time I would have looked for advice on how to quit surgery. How many more days was I going to come home from work physically and emotionally exhausted, before I realised that I had had enough? Around a decade after leaving medical school, everything was finally catching up to me.

I'd had a particularly bad day at work recently. The boss was in a foul mood, and in full flight yelled at everyone who even dared breathe audibly. The ward was full of desperately sick people, some of them clinging on for dear life, and watching them suffer incessantly is taxing. I hadn't slept more than a few hours each night, and exercise and socialising seemed like a distant memory of something someone who looked a little like me used to do. My husband was not really the support I needed, consumed by his own work and at times seeming frustrated with the person I had become. If I saw a patient like me, I would have written them a medical certificate for time off work and sent them to a psychologist for expert help. But I decided to keep pushing on, alone.

It was dark when I got home, not unusual. I was always arriving and leaving when the sun was nowhere to be seen. When I opened the door to my apartment I sobbed, for what seemed like the billionth time that week, washing away some of the exhaustion and pain. All of a sudden my sadness was replaced with rage and I hurled a Chinese cookbook across the living room. Which turned out to be a very bad idea because my left middle finger slammed into the arm of the couch and almost immediately swelled to double its size and morphed into a concerning shade of blue.

I knew I'd broken my finger but, like any good doctor, I took on the role of an awful patient and instead lay on the floor and tried to ignore the pain. By the time I woke up the next day, my whole hand had swollen and I quickly took off my wedding rings before they got stuck. I just avoided becoming a cautionary tale about what not to do when you injure your hand and end up having to have rings cut off in the ED. When I turned up to work, my colleagues all pulled the same face—your finger is very clearly broken and gross, go and deal with it.

There aren't many perks to working in health care but being able to get a quick X-ray when you hurt yourself by throwing a cookbook would be one of them. It turned out everyone was right and I had broken my finger. There were six weeks in a splint ahead of me.

But part of me that day wondered if this was my out from surgery. It was a strange, intrusive thought that I'd shoved down as far as it could go, away from consciousness. But it kept jumping back up. This could be a legitimate reason to leave surgery without being told that I couldn't hack it. Or perhaps more correctly, telling myself that.

For six weeks, I didn't operate. I went home largely on time, spending my days in the hospital doing paperwork and seeing patients on the wards or teaching the junior staff. I would watch operations without being scrubbed, safely removed from the firing line of my irritable bosses. I went out for dinner mid-week because I could guarantee that I would get home in time to keep a restaurant reservation. I lived a semi-normal life. And you know what?

I really liked it.

As my finger healed, the thought that maybe I didn't want it to get better became more frequent. I got curious as to why it was there to begin with. The most obvious reason is that medicine doesn't tolerate quitters. When someone says that they used to be a surgeon, or a surgical trainee, but they left, although we may long for that same freedom, we privately slip into the tired old story that they weren't tough enough or good enough or something else 'enough' and that it's best to weed out the weak as early as possible. A plastic surgeon I was a registrar for used to say exactly this about me when I decided to pursue cardiac surgery; in fact he still says he 'broke me' so badly I had to go and do cardiac surgery instead. It's telling of the culture of medicine that someone would so brazenly say this, like it was an achievement to be proud of.

I sat down at my computer to compose a letter of resignation for the hospital. 'It is with great sadness that I write to you to resign my position.' Except that there wasn't much sadness, there was only relief. My resignation letter turned into something resembling a diary entry in which I detailed all of the broken parts of me, not just my finger, that I felt would never be able to come back together if I stayed in cardiac surgery. I even wrote how I'd broken my middle finger on my left hand, which meant that I was often walking around inadvertently flipping the bird at people as my splint kept my middle finger straight in a silent act of defiance to the system that I felt was breaking me.

And as I finished the letter, I felt this strange sense of renewal. Cardiac surgery, somehow, got a reprieve that day. Even if only out of sheer stubbornness, I decided to tear up my letter (or more accurately, delete it) and carry on. I knew that I could stick it out just long enough to get a consultant job and have some stability in my life. If I left now, I'd have nothing to show for the time I had already served. After just one more year, if I still wished that my finger was broken, I'd have a qualification to show for my time, a qualification that could open doors and serve as a reminder to myself and to others that I could hack the pressure.

The reality was that there were times when I was only just surviving that pressure.

I turned up to work defiant and determined, but not necessarily in a good way. Instead of being quietly backed into a keyboard, when the bosses let fly I would roll my eyes at them and answer back. One of them caught me one day: 'Don't make that face at me!' he yelled.

'I'm not making a face at you; this is just my face.'

I felt strangely like I couldn't be hurt anymore. I do wish I hadn't manifested my defiance in that way; had I channelled that stubbornness into something more positive, I think I could have thrived in that environment rather than felt like a comic book antihero, although I wasn't that either.

I let the darkness consume me and I wish that it hadn't. It's only now, looking back on that time, that I wonder what happened to the stubborn young intern who would have risen to the occasion and been amazing, if only to prove them wrong. What happened to the doctor who would relish the pressure of overly demanding and hyper-critical bosses? I think that there's a rising to exceed expectations that comes from a place of wanting to make you better— and then there's just being ground down by bullshit.

More importantly, it never occurred to me that I shouldn't have to rise to the occasion to prove bullies wrong. Surviving was more of an achievement than thriving in surgery and that is such a fucked-up way of looking at the world.

It wasn't just stubbornness that kept me there. I did still love my job but, in a strange moment of clarity, I knew I loved it just a little less than I once did. Surgery was a bit like swimming in the ocean: you can love the water and you can love the thrill of catching a wave, but every now and again the water will envelop you and try to drown you. Surgery can be wonderful but the nature of the beast is that sometimes in the thrill and the love of what you do, it can feel a little like you're drowning.

It would be nice if the hospitals and the people inside them didn't feel the need to hold your head under.

6

FELLOW

What becomes of the broken-hearted

In all of the angst, I had one very important task ahead of me that would require all of my concentration—my fellowship exams. Just over a year earlier, I had been ready to quit but something made me grit my teeth and make it through this major milestone. For the better part of twelve months, I did nothing except work and study. I had research articles and textbooks on me at all times in case I could steal a moment to study.

Fellowship exams are a huge test, designed to ensure that you have the knowledge and skill to become an independent specialist. They loom large over your entire training, your entire career, in fact, because unless you pass these exams you will not become a consultant surgeon. Not only that, but the exams cost nearly $8000 to sit, and if you fail there is no refund.

Over the course of two days, I answered every question thrown at me about cardiothoracic surgery. I examined patients and told the examiners in great detail how I would manage their cardiac diagnosis; one patient agreed with my management plan and gave me a thumbs-up. After two days, I wasn't sure, but I thought I had done enough to be allowed into the prestigious club.

On the third day, all of us who had sat our exams from every surgical specialty gathered in the lobby of a hotel in Sydney. You could practically smell the anxiety; each and every one of us had come to learn our fate. In order to find out whether the sacrifices of the last year (and before) had been worth it, we were all ushered into a conference room with long tables lined up against one wall. We were told that on command we were to head to the table of our specialty, find the envelope with our candidate number on it and inside would be our result. My heart was pounding so hard.

I had sat my exam with friends, three other men who I had trained and studied with. They were as nervous as I was. I turned to them and said, 'If I disappear, it isn't good news but please don't call me, I'll call you when I feel better.'

At the signal, I raced to the cardiothoracic table and found my number. I retreated outside the conference room for a little bit of privacy away from the crowds to open my letter. *Successful*.

It may sound dramatic, but I fell to the ground, sobbing. There was not a single other event in my life that had brought me such joy and such pride. Through big gulps, I picked up my phone and rang my boss back in Perth, the same one who had stood opposite me through so many surgeries, and wailed into the phone that I had passed.

My friends came out and found me, a heaving, crying mess. They later told me that I was crying so much they thought I had failed. In fairness, if I had looked up through my tears for just a second, I'd have seen I wasn't alone. There were dozens of grown men and women in suits, some with family, all doing the same thing.

'I passed!' I told them. 'It's the best day of my life!' Everything I had given, I thought, was all worth it for this one perfect moment.

***

After my exams, I moved on from my previous hospital, rescued by one of the kindest heart surgeons, who knew I was struggling and was now in the world of paediatric cardiac surgery. When I was a really junior registrar, I had loved paediatric cardiac surgery. Even with the most complex abnormalities that babies can be born with, the surgery to repair them was, in theory at least, perfectly simple by comparison. If the blood goes the wrong way here, you simply patch this hole here and add a tube there. It's poetic but, in practice, it can be unbelievably complex and unforgiving. The heart of a newborn is about the size of a walnut—there is no room for error.

At the kids' hospital, I developed a reputation as a shit magnet. A 'shit magnet' is the clinical term for someone who, whenever they're on call, has everything bad or dramatic happen. In my very first weekend on call, I had an emergency where I had to re-open the chest of a baby not even a week old who had gone into cardiac arrest. After heart surgery, the heart can be prone to electrical issues that lead to unusual and sometimes dangerous heart rhythms. To prevent that and also help us treat the problem, if possible, we sew little wires onto the heart that protrude through the skin, just below the wound, allowing us to give tiny bursts of electricity to the heart, protecting the baby from danger-ous heart rhythms after surgery. Once the danger period for rhythm issues is over we pull them off, simply by pulling them out through the skin. On this occasion, the pulling of the wire caused something to bleed, leading to a condition called tamponade, where the bleeding squashed the heart and sent the baby into cardiac arrest. So here I was, my first week in paediatric cardiac surgery with a full-blown cardiac arrest. I distinctly remember taking a split second to look at the baby and think to myself this was a completely screwed up way to start my life in paediatrics.

For a while, it seemed that every time I walked into the ICU a baby had a problem like this, and the nurses started to joke—but not really—that I was bad luck and should not be allowed in the unit anymore. (Nurses never joke about being a shit magnet, even when it seems like they are. They just want you as far away as possible so you can't cause mischief.)

Given that in the course of a couple of months, I had put several babies on ECMO, re-opened chests or done CPR on kids, I was beginning to think that they were right. Maybe I needed to burn some sage on my Birkenstocks, because clearly they or something else on me was bad karma and those demons needed to be exorcised.

In contrast to the aggressive and jaded culture of an adult hospital, paediatric hospitals are filled with people who by and large are unfailingly lovely. I don't know if it's because people who want to work with children are predisposed to be saintly: working as a team cohesively to help children, perhaps the noblest pursuit there is. Or is it the bright colours, cartoons and uplifting movies like *Frozen* on repeat that means when you work there, you simply can't help but be in a good mood?

Having fun and being happy and entertaining are such a part of a children's hospital that this hospital had an annual dress-up day where staff would come in costumes like super-heroes, Disney stars and favoured nursery rhyme characters. The corridors would be filled with Supermen, Elsas, Storm Troopers and fairies. Staff working in critical care areas, like heart surgery and ICU, were banned from participating because, so the story went, many years ago a child in ICU had died and the bad news had been delivered to the family by a doctor dressed as a clown. I don't know how true that story was, but it was a smart move to have that policy. Neverthe-less, working at the kids' hospital was welcome relief from the ruthless, individualistic, pissing-contest culture that often permeates an adult hospital. And there were no tiny planes and organ retrievals involved.

But as much as I enjoyed the work and adored the people, increasingly I started to find the realities of dealing with really sick kids hard. Day after day, I saw kids who had just had the misfortune of being born with hearts that were not made according to specifications. I started to be bogged down in the unfairness of it all. They had done nothing to deserve this. They had no blame whatsoever to bear and yet sometimes, when they were only minutes old, we were invading their chest to save their lives. Why should someone not even a day old have to fight for their life? Why should the families have to hand over their baby, their most precious creation, to an anaesthetist to drift off to sleep so they can have open-heart surgery when their birth was still a fresh, week-old memory? If you want to see what unfairness looks like, a kids' hospital is the place for that.

CASE 9

Very often, we diagnose heart problems before a baby is even born. When the heart problem is very severe, labour might be induced or a caesarean section performed. Tolerating the sometimes unpredictable nature of labour is not ideal for a baby with a sick heart. We knew this baby was coming. His mum had been told the devastating news that his heart was not right about halfway through her pregnancy. When his heart had been forming, it had switched the two main blood vessels out. This condition, called transposition of the great arteries, meant that when he was born, when his heart and lungs would have to work unaided in the outside world, his body would get oxygen poor blood. Imagine the happiest moments of a first pregnancy, seeing your baby on ultrasound, stolen from you by conversations of how, when only a few days old, your baby would need heart surgery.

We knew baby Michael was on his way to the paediatric ICU, his mother having had a caesarean section in the adult hospital that adjoined us, just up the corridor. He arrived safely but, rather than spending those first few moments of his life cuddled with Mum and Dad, pink and warm, he was descended upon by an army of doctors and nurses trying to stabilise his sick little heart. Michael wasn't just being cared for; we were desperately trying to find out more about his heart using an ultrasound probe that looked nearly as big as he was to try to discover the intricacies of his condition. Michael's heart was more broken than we first thought, like it had been booby trapped for his surgery. It felt like whatever happiness his safe birth had brought was being stolen by mounting bad news.

Michael was just six days old when his mum bundled him into the arms of an anaesthetist to put him to sleep so that we could fix his little heart. Before we started the surgery, we stood around in a team and discussed plan A, then plan B and so on, because this was going to be the most precarious surgery we had performed on a newborn in some time. The mood was sombre and serious, starkly contrasting with the cartoon mermaids and undersea scene painted on the theatre walls.

Hours and hours ticked by and the consultant reached for every trick in the book. He unscrubbed to call colleagues for advice. At one point, there were three consultant surgeons around the table. Michael's little heart was so sick and six hours of surgery hadn't helped it recover like we had hoped it would. He was getting medications through a tube in his neck veins, a central line, to help encourage his heart to muster any force it could and keep this child alive. We could do no more that day and so we covered his chest, leaving the sternum open so that his swollen and bruised heart wouldn't have the added insult of being squashed behind it.

Michael was only back in ICU for a few hours when his heart stopped, and since none of us had been optimistic for anything else we immediately leapt off our chairs that surrounded his tiny cot, opening his chest and gently squeezing his tiny heart between each of our fingers in turn. The internal cardiac massage was to tide him over while we wheeled in the ECMO machine, which can sustain the circulation for days or even weeks. It felt like it took an eternity, but in less than ten minutes Michael's heart was resting and the machine was keeping him alive in the most invasive way possible.

The tiny baby was now embraced by tubes and machines that dwarfed his little body, each utterly necessary to keep him alive. We thought that with the extremely complex problems his heart had, plus hours and hours of surgery, his tiny heart was too injured to work alone. His parents listened intently while they were told that we didn't know what was going to happen but we hoped that, while his heart rested, it might have the chance to recover over the coming days. I could see in the eyes of some of the experienced doctors and nurses that they weren't so sure, but who were we to destroy the hope of this new family?

The days passed, one after the other, almost every one bringing new challenges. There was bleeding and kidney failure or early infections. And while we all worked hard to put out these little spot fires, after nearly two weeks on ECMO as we tried to claw back life for little Michael, one thing never recovered and that was his heart. It was completely unable to do the one thing he needed it to: beat strongly and sustain his little life.

Michael's parents were ushered into a little room by my consultant and the consultant intensive care doctor. The whole ICU knew what was going on behind the closed door of that room, even though we weren't in there. His parents were being told that his heart was too sick, that if it hadn't recovered after two weeks, it was never going to. They were told that he had been given the very best that modern medicine had to offer. They were told that once we switched off the ECMO machine, he would die. They were told that they wouldn't get to go home with their baby.

It's an illusion of choice, when we tell people this kind of news and ask for their permission to turn off the machines that give the perception of life. Because nature and, in this case, disease have made the choice for us all. If any of us had any choice, little Michael would be starting school soon, rather than being the absent older brother his future siblings would be told was an angel in heaven watching over them.

And so, on a Friday afternoon, Michael sat in his parents' arms. The ICU nurses had taken out as many pipes and tubes as possible so that, for one last time, he looked like the baby whom they had wished for. The deception was only given away by the ECMO tubes coming from his chest. The consultant turned off the machine and placed clamps across the tubing, freeing him from ECMO and letting him pass peacefully, untethered from the technology that had ultimately failed to save his life.

He died peacefully and quickly, as his mum and dad held his tiny, broken body and told him that they loved him and that he was perfect. And he was, despite his sick little heart.

I went home that evening, climbing the four flights of stairs to my apartment in the rain. I sat down on that top step, outside my front door, and cried while the raindrops pummelled me. It felt for a moment like my tears were even stronger than the storm. But crying doesn't cut it in moments like this; only numbness feels right because my emotional capacity could never comprehend the unbearable pain that I had just witnessed.

I made the decision that day that I could never be a paediatric heart surgeon. I don't have whatever special quality it takes to face up to that loss, even as a kind of spectator, for the rest of my career. For all the bubbles and cartoons, costumes and camaraderie, nothing would be bright enough to replace that kind of darkness.

After being a registrar most people will become a fellow, a
period of time where you do even more training in a sub-
specialty area. It's kind of like finishing school for surgeons.
Some people travel around the world, some stay locally.
When and where you do your fellowship, for Australian
surgeons at least, seems to be part bragging rights and part
actually learning new and different skills.

I was due to go and get my bragging rights at a UK hospital
but, just before I was gearing up to leave, the NHS slumped
into a deep crisis. Throughout the UK, junior doctors went
on strike after the Tory government proposed changes that
would see the already overworked, understaffed and under-
paid NHS doctors subjected to a significant decline in their
working conditions. The NHS runs on the smell of an oily
rag, delivering world-class care on a minuscule budget. One
of the reasons that this works is that its staff is unbelievably
proud and dedicated, which it seems the government had
taken advantage of for too long.

For me, though, that meant there was no longer any
UK fellowship. No Big Ben, no weekend trips to Spain, no
working with some of the world's most brilliant surgeons
and no bragging rights. I tried to get a fellow job anywhere

I could, but at the eleventh hour, it was unanswered emails or a resounding no everywhere I turned. At the same time, I was trying to juggle my career with my husband's, and although he had initially wanted to spend time in London too he was not even remotely willing to travel to the many opportunities that I presented to him: Canada, the US, other UK cities. It was the first time I felt that despite the fact that my career held a lot more prestige, a lot more earning capacity and had come at much more sacrifice than his, as the wife it would probably still come second.

I decided to be a fellow locally after all of this, finally giving up cold calling every surgeon around the world that I could. I was scared to do this; surgeons who don't go away are always treated like outcasts, like you didn't love your career enough to uproot your life. It was pure and utter surgical snobbery. Just because you go to the Mayo Clinic or a premier European hospital doesn't mean that you get the training of a lifetime. You could spend a year just watching the great professor from the sidelines, but the cachet seemed to be all anyone was after.

My first day at the new hospital as a fellow, I was greeted by an epic Sydney summer storm. As I made my way to the ward to join the team, I dodged buckets and hospital blankets catching water falling from the ceiling. Walking on to the ward, a patient shouted out for help as I walked by, asking for another blanket. A nurse appeared and said that we were all out of blankets because they were being used to mop up the deluge coming through the roof. The door to the office was hanging by a thread, literally, with its handle held on by gaffer tape. This is what happens to hospitals that serve lower socio-economic areas: they're forgotten, left to fall into disrepair without the interest of politicians or celebrity patients to draw huge spending to create shiny new facilities. Health care in Australia might be free for everyone, but it sure as hell isn't equal.

Nonetheless, I had found what I really wanted out of a fellowship year—the opportunity to operate, doing the hard cases with outstanding surgeons who would impart to me years of expertise and wisdom. Without the threat of exams hanging over my head, I could just operate, day in and day out. And as a fellow, not just a registrar, the challenging cases were no longer out of reach; in fact, I was expected to step up and do them. Not only that, I felt that maybe away from the desperate sadness of paediatric cardiac surgery, I could stop coming home from work crying about some terrible unfairness I had just seen.

I may not have travelled around the world, but I got to work with some of the finest surgeons at that hospital and, although I didn't realise it at the time, some of the noblest clinicians I'd ever met. Every other place I'd worked, the consultants were always at each other's throats, just barely disguising their ultra-competitiveness with one another at best or their outright disdain at worst. In this hospital, the bosses were collegiate and supportive of each other in a way I had never really seen before. There were no sexually inappropriate jokes, there was no ass grabbing, there was no bitching about each other behind their backs. Just a group of people there to do the work and support one another in doing that. How had I been missing that everywhere else I had worked?

I don't mean that everything was sunshine and rainbows there. But looking back, I wonder how starved I was for any kind of functional workplace that I even got excited about the dark parts.

'Twenty-four-hour shifts?' I repeated, just making sure I had heard correctly. Turns out I definitely had heard correctly, and all the registrars and fellows were required to do 24-hour shifts, at least once a week. You would do your normal day, operating or seeing patients, and then overnight you would cover the cardiac intensive care unit. I did for a second wonder how 24-hour shifts were actually legal under the industrial agreement but immediately forgot about it, because even if it wasn't allowed, complaining that a roster wasn't lawful would only ever earn you a reputation as a troublemaker and some form of retribution.

I'm pretty adept at being awake for long periods of time. Not regularly; I've never been one of those people who can operate on just four hours' sleep a night. I like sleep and I think I'm a nicer and healthier human when I've had some. But, importantly, I know that when I'm tired and when I have to stay awake, operating into the wee small hours (or beyond), I can do it. As a registrar I pulled some horrific hours, but as much as I hated it I knew it served a purpose. One plastic surgery consultant once told me, 'You need to know how to operate when you're tired because every now and again, you have to. Someone's life will depend on it.' Although he also wisely said that fatigue should not be the norm and we do know that fatigue impairs performance, no matter how 'okay' you think you are.

That's not what this was. This was a classic case of doing something the same way because that's the way it's always been done.

In fairness, a lot of the time you could sneak a few hours' sleep in the ICU. The nurses had a tonne of standing orders—fluids and basic medications that were prescribed in advance, and if a patient needed them they could start them without asking a doctor. As soon as a patient fell outside pre-determined parameters, we changed plans. But probably more importantly, these ICU nurses were the cream of the crop. They were astute and experienced, but they were also compassionate and tried to let us get some rest wherever possible. They were lifesavers in more ways than one.

For the hospital's part, they didn't exactly endorse sleeping while on shift. 'You're not actually being paid to sleep' is a line I've heard in almost every hospital I've ever worked in. Yes, we were all aware of that but, if you want us to be able to do our jobs and to do them well, you'll help us get rest whenever and wherever we can.

About once every six weeks or so, the roster meant that we would have to do a weekend of 24-hour shifts and on call, bundled into one. Which meant working 24 hours on Friday, going home on Saturday morning to get some sleep but also be on call all Saturday, and then doing 24 hours from Sunday morning. The dread that filled me in the lead-up to these weekends is hard to put into words because, in theory, you could get unlucky and have to work a solid 72 hours.

CASE 10

It was about midway through the year before my fears came true. I'd gone home on Saturday, had some sleep and was about to tempt fate by heading out for a short evening run to clear the cobwebs when my phone rang. The hospital number flashed up on the screen. 'Fuck,' I said just loud enough for the lady passing me on the sidewalk to hear (and judge me for), and for some reason I felt that this wouldn't be some simple question that I could answer over the phone. The superstition turned out to be correct: a man who had been stabbed multiple times in the chest, back and abdomen was on his way in.

I tempted the red-light cameras on my way in to the hospital (I have never been pulled over for speeding or other traffic-related offences on my way into an emergency, which is good, since we are not entitled to disregard road rules), and I sprinted through the car park to the ED. The man had been stabbed seven times: three in the chest, twice in the belly and once in the back. The general surgeon would look after the belly and I would deal with the chest. I rang the consultant on call and told him I was going to take this man to theatre to find out what was bleeding. For a consultant the good thing about having a fellow on call is that you have a qualified surgeon who can operate independently. 'Call me if you need me,' he said and hung up. In many hospitals, junior doctors are the real workhorses of the medical teams; from my perspective, it was a love–hate relationship of enjoying the autonomy but also wanting some back up, if only because I had only had a few hours' sleep.

The general surgeon opened the abdomen, making a cut in the middle of the belly from top to bottom. At the same time, I made a cut on the left side of the chest. We chased every stab wound from outside and in, repairing each structure that the knife had encountered. I started sewing up holes in the lung and bleeding vessels in the chest wall. The general surgeon tried to stop the bleeding liver by packing it with surgical swabs and repaired holes in the bowel that, left unchecked, would leak bowel contents through the abdomen and cause overwhelming sepsis. We worked for hours on this man before we could finally close his wounds, both the big ones we had made and the seven smaller wounds from the knife. At the end, though, he was safe and we wearily packed up.

'All done. Lung lacs [lacerations] and chest wall bleeds repaired. Abdo sorted too,' I texted my boss, referring to the lung lacerations I had sewn shut. No sooner had the text flown off into the ether than things took a turn for the worse.

The anaesthetist shouted out, 'Guys, something's wrong. Nikki, I think he has a tension pneumothorax,' as I rushed to the left chest where I had been operating. I grabbed a stethoscope and listened as air rushed in and out of the left side: no indications of a collapsed lung. I swapped the stethoscope to the right chest where I was met with silence. The right lung was collapsed, air collecting around the right lung pushing on the heart and the right lung causing his breathing to struggle and his heart to labour under the extra pressure.

The scrub nurse had heard someone say 'pneumothorax' and pre-emptively got me a chest drain. Those kinds of manoeuvres, anticipating shit hitting the fan, save lives. I plunged the scalpel into the right side of his chest and pushed a surgical forcep into the chest, where air hissed out at me, and I followed that by inserting a tube about the size of my index finger. I should have known better than to tempt fate and text the boss before the patient was safely off the operating table and not a moment sooner.

Before I left the hospital, I had to do an important piece of paperwork—fill in an overtime form so that I actually got paid for the six hours of work I had just done. I always feel uncomfortable claiming money for doing this, partly because for years I have a sense of duty to do good but also because I'd listened to senior doctors or administrators admonish us for claiming overtime, guilt-tripping us by saying that the system was always stretched and we shouldn't want to add to that burden. It was drilled into us from an early age that we were supposed to love this so much, we'd virtually (and actually) do it for free. Especially on a weekend, once you go over a certain time cap, the rates that I have to be paid are high and, although I wasn't breaking laws or even being paid unreasonably for the responsibility I had just shouldered, I couldn't shake that I should feel ashamed for wanting to be compensated.

In that hospital, in order to get paid overtime, you had to fill in your overtime sheet, with the patient's details and why it was such a necessity for you to be there. You then had to sign a declaration that you were genuinely required to be there and that you had also tried to ensure that you had tidied up any other work that might happen, lest you had to go back and cost the hospital even more money for an emergency.

Once you had done that, you had to find the after-hours director of nursing, the most senior nurse in the hospital, who would sign your overtime form to confirm that you were not a dirty, dirty liar. Like she had nothing better to do than sign paperwork for doctors. The director of nursing was responsible for overseeing crucial operations for nurses for the entire hospital but by all means let's interrupt her. I chased her around four wards before I found her to give her seal of approval, where we were both equally annoyed at having to do superfluous nonsense like this.

Trustworthy enough to do emergency surgery on a trauma patient. Not trustworthy enough to accurately declare how long I was in the hospital so I could get paid for that work.

CRITICAL REFLECTION QUESTION
What do you observe about the life of a cardiothoracic fellow in this case study?

That's medicine for you—we can treat you like crucial and respected members of the workforce one minute, the next we will dehumanise you as much as possible. For a humanistic profession, I was beginning to discover just how lacking in humanity it could be for the people who work in it.

* * *

One of the best parts of this job for me was treating some of the most interesting and challenging illnesses I had ever seen. The hospital was situated in the heart of one of the lowest socio-economic areas in town. I've always been very proud of Australia's free healthcare system, where if you need treatment you will get it, but I had erroneously lulled myself into believing that, because of that, money doesn't matter as much here when it comes to your health. I was wildly mistaken. Some days in this hospital felt like I was practising medicine in a totally different and far less affluent country than Australia.

In my entire career, I had never seen so many people with advanced cancer or advanced heart disease. They would stay at home, knowing something was wrong but feeling unable to come and seek help. Many were working to support entire extended families. Some came from immigrant backgrounds with a fear of being neglected in hospitals, or they were just absolutely petrified. Meaning that, by the time they came to us, they were some of the sickest patients I had ever seen. It all started to fall into place for me: this was an area where celebrity backers aren't around and the aggressive, critical judgement of more affluent people isn't there to scream loudly for better standards. And as a result, the hospital ceiling threatened to collapse in the rain, with not enough blankets to soak up the puddles and warm the patients in one of the sickest and most neglected portions of our community.

One such patient was Jim. Jim had worked as a bricklayer until he was just 40, when a back injury at work meant that physical labour was no longer an option, and he was forced on to welfare—probably for the rest of his life. About a year before he came to the hospital, diabetes and a motorcycle accident had meant that Jim's left leg had to be amputated above the knee, leaving him relegated to a wheelchair. Despite his seemingly terrible fortune, Jim was a salt-of-the-earth character, warm and lovely even in the face his constant stream of difficulties.

Jim had been sick for a week by the time he came to hospital, short of breath and a bit nauseous. Over time, diabetes had destroyed his nerves, meaning that he couldn't feel the pain of the big heart attack he was having. His blood sugars were wildly out of control, nearly three times what they should have been, which eventually prompted his daughter to force him to hospital. Jim, despite his sunny outlook, hated hospitals. Which was understandable; the last time he had been admitted to hospital, he had lost a leg, the diabetes causing his injured left leg to succumb to overwhelming infection. Jim had all the reasons in the world to want to stay away from people like me but now he had no choice.

Jim's heart was badly damaged by the heart attack, which had affected a branch of the right coronary artery to the point where there was nothing anyone could do for it. If Jim had felt pain early on and come straight to hospital, we might have saved that section of his heart. The other two big coronary arteries were still open—but only just. There was much discussion between one of my consultants and the cardiologists about what we could do for Jim. If we left him, he was at risk of another heart attack that would finish off the rest of his heart and Jim in the process. If we operated on him, he was very high risk for all kinds of problems: dying during surgery, pneumonia, infections, kidney failure, the list went on. In the end, though, my boss made the tough call—Jim would need surgery.

Jim was jovial all the way to the operating theatre and I chatted to him while he went off to sleep. Just before the anaesthetist gave him the propofol, the medication to make him unconscious, his jovial mask slipped as he looked to the ceiling to say to all of us, 'Take care of me, please,' as the mask was placed over his face and he drifted off to sleep. With him safely in the land of oblivion, the theatre bustled, with everyone doing their bit to get him ready for surgery. A urinary catheter went in, the anaesthetist put in a central line and we performed a team time-out.

'This is Jim,' I read off his name band, reciting his medical record number and date of birth from the hospital band on his right (and only) ankle. 'Consented for coronary artery bypass grafting with LIMA and vein, signed and dated. Antibiotics, blood?' I asked the anaesthetist. 'Yep, two grams cephazolin and cross-match is in the room,' he answered. Our scrub nurse finished it off, asking if anyone had any questions. 'Great!' I said cheerfully, just as the boss walked in.

At the scrub sink, we stood chatting about what we were going to do. He was taking this case, rather than me. Jim was too sick and generally when the stakes were high, the consultant is the one doing all of the operating. Despite the fact that I was well and truly capable of doing this surgery, when the odds are stacked against us we want our most experienced operator, because with people like Jim the tiny margin for error is even smaller. I was going to be taking the vein from Jim's remaining right leg to use to bypass one of the remaining blocked arteries, again because we wanted the most senior person available. This wasn't a leg that we wanted people learning or practising on; Jim needed every chance we could give him. And he was in brilliant hands; this boss was (and remains) one of my absolute favourite people to work with. He was calm, controlled and experienced; I wish I had told him back then how much I appreciated working for him.

Jim's operation went surprisingly smoothly given how sick he was coming into the surgery. It was old-school heart surgery: nothing fancy, nothing new, just a good, quick operation. His heart was not perfect, but with the addition of two brand new bypasses it was significantly happier, beating away much more strongly than we could have hoped for.

With Jim safely off bypass, the boss left me and one of our registrars to close up and finish the case. I started inspecting everywhere we had cut for bleeding—the underside of the sternum, the bypass grafts—and as I looked at the aorta, where the saphenous vein had been plugged into to take blood to the blocked coronary artery, a little jet shot up at me.

'6-0 thanks!' I said as I put a little square of gauze on the vessel (called a 'top-end') so that I didn't get blood on my loupes, obscuring my vision. The scrub nurse placed the needle holder in my hand, loaded with a fine suture that I then plunged into the margin where the vein met the aorta. And then, as I usually did, I snapped the needle off the string to give back to her before I tied the suture. Although I usually did it, I really shouldn't have, because when you snap the needle off like that it can jump off and get lost.

Which is exactly what happened that day.

'Oh, shit! I'm so sorry, where did it go?' I asked as I tied down the suture. Every single item must be accounted for at the end of an operation and a lost needle is just not acceptable. With the suture tied, we started looking everywhere for the lost needle. I was so annoyed with myself for being too impatient to wait for someone to get scissors and cut the needle off. To ensure that it hadn't landed back in Jim's chest, we had to perform an X-ray in theatre. This is a frustrating thing about losing something in a heart operation: while everyone is trying to locate the missing item, our attention is diverted, focusing on finding whatever it is we've lost rather than continuing with the operation.

In heart surgery, we sometimes use literally hundreds of tiny needles, dozens of gauze swabs and more instruments than you have ever seen in your life. Things do go missing, maybe once a week or a fortnight, but they are always located. This day, though, the needle was nowhere to be found. I'd even taken off my shoes to make sure it hadn't landed in one of them. The portable X-ray in theatre confirmed that Jim's chest was not harbouring the wayward needle. Jim's chest still needed closing, so with certainty that the 6-0 needle wasn't in there, I closed his chest and placed his dressings on. Out of the corner of my eye, I could see the nurse in charge of our theatre circling me like a buzzard over a dead body. The scrub nurse and I were about to get yelled at for losing a needle. In fairness, I deserved it.

Just as the drapes came off, the scrub nurse yelled out, 'I got it!' as she reached into the jug of fluid on her trolley. How I had managed to flick that tiny needle from the table to land perfectly in the jug of fluid more than a metre away I will never know. Finding the needle only meant good things; both the scrub nurse and I were off the hook. And of course, importantly, it was not inside Jim.

Although Jim's operation had gone well, he struggled after surgery. All in all, he spent four nights asleep in ICU as we fought to stabilise his sick heart and his kidneys. He developed pneumonia while he was on the ventilator, meaning that we had to bomb his body with antibiotics and medicines to keep his blood pressure up and help his heart beat stronger. About four days after his surgery, the wound on his leg started to look infected.

Diabetes is really a true enemy of the surgeon and patient alike. Years of diabetes damage our nerves, our blood vessels and our immune cells, meaning that infection can be a constant threat in situations like this. The bad blood supply and sub-optimal immune system mean that bacteria can run rampant in a wound like the one Jim had on his remaining leg. We had tried to keep the infected wound under control on the ward but after a week he needed an operation to cut away the dead and infected tissue, called debridement, to give it the best chance of healing. The registrars booked everything, got Jim to sign a consent form and he was in theatre the next day.

After Jim's debridement, I ran into the registrar who was on the case with the boss. 'How did it go?' The registrar just rolled his eyes and shook his head. Oh no, I thought, Jim's only leg. 'The wound wasn't too bad actually, it should heal nicely. But before his surgery—what a pain in the arse!'

In surgeries that happen on a side, the left or right, there is a tonne of checkpoints in the surgical journey to ensure that the correct side is operated on. And with good reason: people have had surgeries on the wrong knee or lost the wrong kidney, sometimes with devastating consequences. One of the things we do is mark the side, using a big sharpie and an arrow to indicate to everyone which is the correct side.

'We went to get Jim around to theatre but they wouldn't let him leave holding bay [the large communal room where patients await their surgery before actually going into theatre]. They called me and told me that they couldn't let him go because he wasn't marked, so, of course, I went around there to mark him when it dawned on me that he didn't need his leg marked. He only has one leg; it's physically impossible to operate on the wrong leg!' I started laughing, knowing full well where this conversation was going.

'I went around there,' he continued, 'and I found the nurse and explained to him that Jim didn't need his leg marked for surgery because he only has one leg so can he please go to theatre now because we're all waiting on him.' As I had predicted, the nursing staff had refused, saying that his leg must be marked because it's policy. My registrar and the nurses had argued for a while before he'd thrown his hands up in defeat and drawn a big arrow on his one and only leg.

'You know, by the time you argued with them, you could have just drawn the arrow and it would have been done with?' I asked him through laughter, imagining the scenario. 'Yeah, but it was wrong. And I'm sick of being a slave to bullshit protocols.' My laughter dried up pretty quickly.

'Yeah, I know, there are so many protocols here for ridiculous unimportant reasons. And so many of them make our jobs harder, not easier, and I certainly don't know if they actually help patients. Getting the correct side is obviously vital, it's inexcusable to fuck that up'—he nodded along—'so I know why everyone was upset.' Although I agreed—Jim had one leg and it was impossible to get the wrong side— it wasn't worth the fight even if on the surface it seemed unnecessary.

As I walked away, I was pleased that Jim's leg was on the mend. But I started to think about the fight my registrar had had. Surgeons hate policy—we feel unnecessarily bound by it. Many policies have arisen for good reasons: to keep patients safe. But many policies exist because of an unwavering obsession that hospitals have for doing things a certain way because they've always been done a certain way, in the face of scientific evidence or feedback that these practices actually keep us from doing our jobs safely and effectively.

Year after year, I felt less inclined to fight useless status quos because nothing ever changed except for my ever-soaring blood pressure. But, equally, the longer I spent in the health system the more frustrated I was by the perpetual red tape, flawed policies and the dehumanisation of a workforce that is at the coalface of some of the most human experiences we could face. When the extreme stresses of saving a life are compounded by existing in an environment that frustrates then breaks any resilience you have left, how can we possibly go on?

7

CONSULTANT SURGEON

To mend a broken heart

I am one of those people who can grind through pretty much anything as long as I know that there is an end in sight, an ultimate goal to work for. And to me, that goal was becoming a consultant surgeon, a fully fledged surgeon. After all, even with deviations in my pathway, I *had* wanted to be a heart surgeon since I was eight years old.

Towards the end of my training, though, it felt like everything was a bit of a struggle. With every passing year, I felt this growing disillusionment. I know that it had all always been there—the sexism, the system that buckles if a butterfly flaps its wings, the suffering of others, the chronic lack of sleep—but the more senior I became in medicine, the more I noticed it all and the more it all bothered me. And when I realised that, as a junior doctor, a mere cog in the vast machine of a hospital (or so I was told), I couldn't fix these problems, it made it hard to soldier on.

To me, though, getting to the pinnacle, to that goal I had set myself so long ago of being a consultant surgeon, let me do two things. The first and most important was to do what I love, because I was still utterly smitten with the heart and I loved nothing more than fixing it for my patients. Even the filthy underbelly of surgery couldn't erase that, I thought. The second reason was that I thought that as a consultant I would finally be in a position to do something about all the things that had frustrated me over the years.

When operations were cancelled because of inefficiencies in the system, I could use my voice that would now hold some authority, some gravitas, to try to advocate for my patients. I would be able to stand proudly in front of a room full of women who wanted to do surgery and show them that I had done it and so they could too. Even from an entirely selfish standpoint, I wouldn't have to feel like the odds were stacked against me. That I wasn't being beaten at every turn, that I had earned my spot by standing strong over the years and passing every test that had been put to me, official and unofficial.

It wasn't just the formal tests that I had to pass. I had to be deemed worthy by those on high and also be in the right place at the right time. Consultant surgeons tend to stay in their jobs until the day they die, no matter how ineffectual they are at their jobs. The cushy public sector pays them well, even if they put in the bare minimum of effort in their positions with very little recourse (or desire) to correct behaviour, especially late in their careers. We used to joke that the only way to get a position was to wait for someone to die or retire.

And then, of course, you have to be tapped on the shoulder by someone in a position of power. Getting a consultant job was not necessarily about being the best, but being deemed to be good enough. And what constituted good enough might mean anything from being a good surgeon to being unlikely to threaten the lucrative private practice of your colleagues.

I had moved back to my hometown after my marriage disintegrated. My marriage ended unceremoniously, although it had been on life support for some time, and I wanted to come back to the familiarity that a hometown can bring and just get on with my life, focusing on my career and finding enjoyment in that once more. I had always sought solace in work when my personal life went to shit. I waited for my tap on the shoulder to step up as a consultant that, at one point, I had been convinced would never come. Especially not after I accidentally received an email not intended for me from the professor of my unit who had written that I was 'fragile' after my divorce and probably 'needed to go elsewhere'. It was the first and last time in my life that I had been called fragile. I also wasn't too fragile to do all of his operating while he—well, I don't know what he did.

When I was finally anointed as a consultant, it felt as though all of my frustrations and criticisms of the system and, at times, the people who worked in it just melted away. Finally, I was going to be able to do the actual job that I felt born to do. Finally, I was going to be able to make a difference in my patients' lives and, maybe, if I was able to change everything that was difficult and broken in surgery, for far more people than my patients.

CASE 11

The operating theatre is kept cold (to cool the patients' core body temperature to protect their organs while they are on bypass), so much so that, as you open the door, the air is almost icy as it hits your face. The lights are bright, and everything is clean and stark. It sounds like a cruel and emotionless place but, for me, it is my sanctuary.

My patient had just been wheeled into theatre, buried under three blankets to keep him warm while the anaesthetists prepared him for surgery. I walked over and grabbed his hand. Since in the fear of what's to come and because with scrub hats and masks familiar faces often get lost, I said, 'It's Dr Stamp here, Phil, how are you?'

Phil laughed at me and said, 'I knew it was you! Now tell me, did you get a good night's sleep last night?' It's a common joke made by nervous patients to break the ice and surreptitiously ask if we're all on our A game. I reassured him, saying we actually cancelled our big party last night just for him. When the jokes subside, sometimes if you look closely you can see a moment of pleading in the eyes, as if to say, 'Please, take care of me,' which I meet with a silent squeeze of the hand to say, 'Of course we will.'

Heart surgery is about as big an operation as you can get. It's so invasive, not just because of the cut I was about to leave down the length of his sternum, but because we are cutting into and stopping a heart: it's like a person's very essence, their soul, is being attacked. Commensurate with this invasiveness comes a cast of thousands: two consultant anaesthetists, an anaesthetic registrar and an anaesthetic technician were there to drift our patients off to sleep and monitor every vital organ function—the heart, the lungs, the brain, the kidneys—throughout the operation. The heart–lung bypass machine was being prepared in the background, going through a series of final checks to ensure everything was in working order, like a plane about to take off. The captain of that plane, the perfusionist, was finetuning the machine, ready to incorporate all the feedback the machine and I gave them so that the operation was indeed possible.

The nurses, three of the most experienced scrub nurses in the hospital, were getting ready as well, opening trays of shiny, sterile instruments, counting not only each instrument but every screw and every tiny component that we needed so they could all be accounted for at the end of the surgery. I had one of my favourite nurses in theatre today, even though I know full well you're not supposed to play favourites. She earned that status not only because I'd known her since I was a baby registrar, but also because she was absolutely excellent at her job. She often knew what instrument I wanted even before I did and she was a fun and amazing colleague (meaning she would sing along to my questionable music choices with me). This team, in particular, had spent so much time together, for so many years, that it felt more like family. And I was as loyal to this family as I was to my own blood relatives. It felt so special to have been with these people since I had been just starting out in my career in surgery to being back here now, this time at the helm. The warmth of my feelings towards them all, to my patient and to these staff members, balanced out the icy-cold air in theatre.

It takes some time for the anaesthetists to work their magic for major surgery. Once the patient is asleep (although it is a state more mysterious than sleep), as it also has to stop the body's natural response to pain and to render it still, the anaesthetist places a plethora of things to monitor the patient's artificial slumber or to give medications and lifesaving concoctions.

For most heart surgeries, the patient gets no fewer than three or four invasive lines to watch over them carefully. They get an arterial line, a tiny plastic tube in the radial artery in the wrist that gives us blood pressure readings in real time; a central venous catheter (called a CVC), placed in one of the jugular veins in the neck that reads the pressure inside the heart and allows us to give medications to increase or decrease the blood pressure, make the heart pump stronger or give fluids and blood if needed; a urinary catheter, a tube placed in through the urethra to the bladder for the dual purpose of dealing with urine, since the patient can't go to the toilet, obviously, but also allows us to watch how much wee someone is making, a key marker of how well the kidneys are going during the surgery. Kidneys are like canaries in coalmines: they're exquisitely sensitive to any little ups and downs in the body's function and often serve as an early warning if something is awry or a beautiful reassurance when things are good.

This whole process can take up to 45 minutes or an hour, depending on the speed and experience of the anaesthetist and how sick the patient is. The anaesthetic registrars, just like the surgical registrars, have to learn these important skills so tend to take a little longer than their bosses. Some of my colleagues use this time to rant that they're taking too long and complain loudly to anyone who will listen. Others use this time to sleep in, rolling into the operating theatre late when they overestimate how long the anaesthetists will need, a habit I find personally unacceptable. For me, this is the pre-game and we should all be there for the pre-game.

I never thought I had a pre-game ritual but, in actual fact, I do. I eat, because it will be several hours before I'll get the chance again and a surgeon with low blood sugar and an audibly rumbling stomach is not conducive to a good operation. I have a pre-game toilet break for the same reasons because, if you need to pee mid-operation, too bad. Once we start, we can't and don't stop. And, most importantly, I use the time to go through everything—tests, imaging, surgery plans—one last time so that by the time I make the incision on the chest, I've already done the operation in my head several times over.

I had two registrars as assistants that day: the first was our trainee, on his way to a career as a cardiac surgeon. He's diligent and gifted and one of my favourite companions in theatre. Not just because he's good at banter, essential in my books, but also because I trust the skills he brings to the table. I knew that, like me, he'd probably looked at the angiogram dozens of times, the echocardiogram even more. I knew that, like me, he'd probably thought of every eventuality, even to the point of causing extraordinary anxiety, which sometimes means I need to tell him to 'stop stressing'. Sometimes I look at him and I'm reminded of my own time in his shoes and then equally astonished that the tables have turned and I'm now the teacher. I'd never call myself the master, though; I hated it when my seniors did that, as if the junior person had nothing to contribute when the reality is that we're here as a team.

My other registrar also happened to be my friend and she has a natural gift and dexterity for surgery. Whenever I showed her a new skill, she picked it up much faster than most of her colleagues. The sad thing for her was that the head of our department seemed to dislike her intensely, disproportionate to anything she had ever done to warrant such an opinion. And as a consequence, he once pulled me aside to tell me that I was being 'too nice' to the registrars. I obliged and kept my distance, which meant a week later he told me not to be too 'stand-offish' with them. More bullshit and playground nonsense to complicate my day.

The anaesthetists were finally ready and every one of us had done our standard pre-operative checks individually: the formal ones (like counting instruments) and informal (pre-game pee) alike. Before we actually started, we had one final check, the team time-out. Everyone stopped what they were doing and checked that we had the right patient, that they had consented for the right operation, that we were operating on the correct side and that we had everything we needed: equipment, blood to transfuse and test results. One big advantage of heart surgery is that there is only one heart; there's no left or right to choose from.

Our final safety check done, I had to get dressed for surgery, putting on my final pieces of armour before heading into battle the enemy threatening Phil's heart. A mask, operating loupes and a headlight that I tightened over my Teenage Mutant Ninja Turtles scrub cap. This is why I have neck pain most days: staring downwards with a whole bunch of stuff weighting down my head is not a natural way for a human neck to function. Most importantly, before I scrubbed into surgery, which I affectionately call 'washing my paws', we needed to select some music. I flicked through Spotify, looking for a playlist that was uplifting and inoffensive, which meant I usually landed on '80s or '90s music.

I inquired to the room, "80s or '90s today, team?' and was met with more requests for '90s than '80s so that's what we got. Heart surgery is serious, but I love music because it helps me concentrate. And, importantly, I love something upbeat because I think that work should be at least a little bit fun, especially when it's so serious. Fittingly for my yearning for fun, Aqua's 'Barbie Girl' came on over the speaker.

The music still tinkled in the background and I sang along as I painted Phil from his neck to his toes in Betadine, an antiseptic to murder any would-be bacterial assassins that might infiltrate the wounds and cause an infection. We then carefully placed sterile drapes that exposed only Phil's chest, legs and his left arm. It's a ritual that I do the exact same way every single time. It has to be perfect, laid on him in a way that's just so. I once had a boss tell me that if he couldn't trust me to get the drapes on correctly, how the hell would he ever trust me to do anything else correctly? Which he said as he was pulling the drapes off to do it all over again because I had, in my inexperience, placed the drape incorrectly across the neck.

The dancing subsided as the moment when I took a scalpel in my hand drew nearer. Like everything else, this was a ritual. I used the handle of the scalpel to press into the skin, leaving a shallow indent at the top, middle and bottom of the sternum, and then used a string to join the dots, leaving a perfectly straight line. I despise crooked wounds with such a passion. It's all the patient has to see of our work. When I was a medical student, a general surgeon once told me that, even though it seems like the least skilful, least exciting or least important part of the operation, it must be perfect. He told me, 'You could leave a boot inside someone, but if they see your wound and think it's perfect, they're going to thank you because they will think the inside is perfect too.' I'd add to that that everything, absolutely everything, should be perfect.

I took the scalpel and followed my line, layer by layer revealing the sternum. The sternal saw glided effortlessly through the bone and splayed it apart. The pericardium houses the heart, the last line of defence, and I broke through that too, showing the heart rocking away inside, never meant to be on display like this. Phil's heart stared back at me and a little part of me was invigorated all over again by this wondrous display of the human body.

Heart surgery is a team sport. Each one of the cast of thousands has a very important job to do. One registrar is operating on Phil's left wrist, carefully harvesting the radial artery, and the other makes a cut on his right leg, to show the saphenous vein. At the same time, I've elevated the left side of Phil's sternum to show the internal mammary artery. Bit by bit, each of us liberates these vessels, borrowing them from their old home to use in the heart, where they will take healthy blood around the blockages in Phil's coronary arteries that gave him a heart attack six weeks ago. I sometimes look at the massive team who all work so hard just for this one surgery and I feel bad when people like Phil sing my praises alone. 'Thank you, Dr Stamp, so much for saving my life,' or words to that effect make me feel icky since this is not a solo pursuit. Not all of my colleagues share in this embarrassment; in fact, they'll take thanks even when they did nothing at all.

'Retractor, please,' I asked my scrub nurse. She's the senior nurse in theatre and, while she is very good at her job, she makes no bones about playing favourites with the surgeons or the nurses. In our close-knit family of heart warriors, she felt like the odd one out, lacking the warmth and collegiality that everyone else possessed in spades. I was not nor was I ever going to be one of her favourites, which means I was persistently on the receiving end of little barbs from her. Like handing me the retractor that I don't use.

Surgeons are adept at performing surgery with all kinds of instruments in the many iterations they are made in. We have to be, because sometimes there is a reason for picking one pair of forceps over another: it's better for a particular job. But, sometimes, there are instruments that we use simply because we like them better, a personal preference. When I have the tools I know and am comfortable with, surgery becomes even more autonomous than usual. And when things just flow, without the interruptions of having to use something you're not comfortable with, it's good for the patient.

The scrub nurse handed me the retractor. I went to put it between the two halves of the sternum to reveal the heart underneath, turning the handle like a car jack that slowly cranks the bone apart. But the retractor was broken, as instruments can be with wear and tear, and instead of holding open the busted retractor slammed shut, nearly catching my finger in the process. And, obviously, also failing at its one job.

I pulled the retractor out, handed it back to the nurse and told her that it was broken. 'I really don't want to lose a finger!' I explained to her.

She took it out of my hand and turned the handle a few times. 'Looks all right now,' she said, and handed it back to me.

Theatre nurses are knowledgeable about the intricacies of the instruments we use—where to find them, how to put

them together, how to fix them when they inevitably break—
and so I tried it again. And again the same thing happened.

'I really can't use this, can you open another retractor for
me, please?' and requested my retractor of choice. She snatched
the retractor from me and said, 'Mr Curmudgeon [not his real
name] used this yesterday and it was fine,' suggesting that the
issue was not with the retractor but rather with me. After a bit
of begging and pleading, my favourite nurse, who was circulating and responsible for retrieving instruments as we needed
them throughout the surgery, returned with what I needed.
I could feel the chill in the air, not from the cool room but
from the judgement from my scrub nurse as she handed it to
me. I felt so small, like I had been not only demoted to uned-
ucated peasant who didn't know what she was doing but also
exposed as a diva, as if requesting instruments that worked
and that suited the patient (and my needs) was like insisting
that someone rub my feet while I operated.

The retractor drama over, I refocused and tried to repress
thoughts about how much my nurse hated me and how
everyone must think I'm shit. The operation trundled along,
although I am never aware of the time. As I zoned in on what
I was doing, my mind on nothing else, I was in my happy
place. There was something so therapeutic, hand-sewing Phil's
radial artery or his internal mammary artery to a coronary
artery, just a millimetre or two wide, with a suture that is not
much thicker than a human hair. This is one of the reasons
the operating theatre is my sanctuary, because doing this and
doing it well brings some strange form of calm to me. It's why

I imagine other people garden or take up pottery. My happy place is sewing minuscule structures together on the surface of someone's heart. Nothing at all odd about that.

The operation went smoothly and I sat down to type up my operation report. I took a moment to look around the room and I felt this deep sense of pride. I was proud of my registrars who were coming along in leaps and bounds; I was proud to be working beside people I'd worked alongside since I was just a baby surgeon with nothing but dreams of one day being at the helm of an operation like this. I was even proud of myself. It had been no easy road to get here, and despite the fact that I found a deep satisfaction and solace in what I do, it was an enormous responsibility.

I was also struck by how much this place felt like home. There's a certain ease and comfort that I get inside an operating theatre: the cool air, the beeps of machines, the hustle and bustle of the team, the sense of purpose and achievement. Its walls insulate me from the unimportant demands and aimless protocols that seem to consume life outside of that room. This is the good place; at least, in my mind, it's supposed to be.

But as I went home that evening, all I could think about was that fucking retractor.

CRITICAL REFLECTION QUESTION
What do you observe about the life of a cardiothoracic surgeon in this case study?

I was enjoying my weekend, amazingly not at work. I was actually on a day off—although with heart surgery, there isn't truly ever a day off. Phone calls or text messages still come through, asking questions or keeping you updated on your patients. Sometimes, you get called in to operate for an emergency or because one of your patients has an issue. Whatever the case, I was never far from my phone. The only time that my phone was really turned off was when I was on a plane, a brief, sweet respite.

The other reason I'd get messages was when something big was happening at work. I think because we're all borderline obsessed with our jobs, we like to be kept abreast of anything and everything that's happening, whether it involves us or not.

'There's a 40-year-old woman going on to ECMO. Massive LMCA infarct,' read the message from my registrar.

There are three main coronary arteries that supply blood to the heart: the right coronary artery, and the left main coronary artery (abbreviated to the LMCA), which divides into two other branches called the left anterior descending and left circumflex. The left main supplies blood to two-thirds of the heart, and when a heart attack involves blockage of that artery it's nicknamed the 'widow maker', since it can wipe out most of your heart very quickly and result in certain death.

A young woman really shouldn't be having a heart attack so big that her heart fails so badly that she needs ECMO, where the patient is connected to a long-term heart-lung machine. ECMO is the crème de la crème of life support, taking over the work of the heart almost entirely.

It turned out that the woman had a condition called spontaneous coronary artery dissection (SCAD), which tends to happen in young women. The inner lining of the artery just tears spontaneously for reasons we don't quite understand. When this happened, it fully blocked the blood supply to the entire left side of her heart. She was absolutely fine when all of a sudden she felt faint and sweaty and immediately knew that something was terribly wrong. Her husband threw her in the back of the car, not wanting to chance it for an ambulance (while it turned out to be a good call in this situation, I'd never normally advise this) and, as they pulled up at the hospital, not even five minutes away, her heart stopped. The ED flew into action and, happily, a short burst of CPR got her circulation going again. But what she really needed was her heart fixed so she was raced to the cardiac catheter lab, where heart diagnostics and emergency stents are done, where they tried to treat the massive heart attack.

The cardiologists worked for hours trying to open up her blocked artery but were unable to. And her heart was limping the whole time, barely able to carry on and sustain life. One of my colleagues was called in to place her on ECMO, just in the nick of time too. As he arrived, her heart stopped again and so he opened her chest and placed the pipes in the heart, having the machine stepping in and saving her life in a matter of minutes. Despite this, things didn't look good. Her heart was severely damaged and only time would tell if it would make a recovery.

On Monday morning, I went to see her in ICU. She was being kept asleep with a combination of medications to make her unconscious, take away pain and stop her from moving: partly to stop her accidentally waking and dislodging the lifesaving equipment she was attached to and partly to keep the body as quiet as possible. When our body is doing less, it takes stress off the heart so that it doesn't have to work so hard. Her heart had not recovered much in the last two days, and the consensus among the dozens of expert doctors who were taking care of her was that in a week or so, if her heart was still so damaged, we'd need to start talking about mechanical hearts and transplants. But it turned out she wasn't going to last that long: her situation deteriorated that morning and we made the decision that she was going to get a mechanical heart that afternoon.

One of my other colleagues and I took her to the operating theatre to insert a mechanical heart. When I first started heart surgery these machines were the size of dinner plates, powered by pipes the size of a hose that emerged from the abdomen, just below the rib cage, and connected to a power console, affectionately known as the 'shopping trolley', that the patient would need to push around. This machine, called an LVAD (left ventricular assist device), had now shrunk down so it comfortably sat in the palm of my hand. The machine is basically a pump; we cut out a piece of the left ventricle muscle the size of a bottle cap and attach the pump, which sucks blood out and sends it to the aorta through another pipe, supplementing the broken heart. A small power cord, called a drive line, connects the pump with the outside world, emerging through the belly where it connects to a battery pack that powers the device, 24 hours a day, uninterrupted.

One of the really interesting things about an LVAD is that people who have one don't have a pulse. When our hearts beat normally, the heart squeezes blood out and then relaxes to fill up again, rhythmically. It's why we have a heartbeat and a pulse. When you feel your pulse, at your wrist or in your neck, each push against your finger represents the whoosh of blood your heart has just pushed out. When I place my stethoscope on your chest, I can hear the rhythmic 'lub-dup' of every heart-beat (the sounds actually come from the valves of the heart snapping shut). In contrast, an LVAD flows continuously, like a pool pump, constantly pushing blood forwards. It means that there is no intermittent pulse, no whoosh against your finger. Someone with an LVAD has no pulse. And when you listen to their heart, the stethoscope hears only the hum of a machine.

All of this happened without her knowledge; her husband had to make the call to give us permission to do this while her life hung in the balance. Imagine that, waking up with a machine inside you, whirring away to keep you alive. It's so hard to fathom, losing days while your body betrays you and is kept alive by a series of surgeries and endless cocktails of lifesaving medications. When you awaken and understand what has happened, it must be unbelievably confronting to know that life has changed irrevocably.

A few days after she woke, Judy had accumulated a large amount of fluid around her left lung. It is a very common occurrence after this surgery; the heart failure and the operation itself irritate the chest, and as a result fluid accumulates around the left lung. It makes breathing a little challenging and the only way to manage it is to put a tiny drain in to let it out.

This was one of the first times I had spoken to Judy when she was fully awake. The blur of the medications to make her sleep and the confusion of this situation meant that I had met her many, many times in a completely one-sided fashion. But on that day, she was fully alert as I told her I was going to need to put a tube in her chest.

There are no two ways about it: having a chest drain really hurts. Even with a lot of local anaesthetic and heavy-duty painkillers, these things are unpleasant. I explained to her what I was going to do and started painting the back of her left chest with antiseptic and making small talk about how she was doing. I'd probably done hundreds of these drains by this stage of my career, so much so that I could probably do them while reciting Shakespeare, they were that familiar to me. But it hurt her. It hurt a lot, and for months afterwards, every time I saw her, Judy would give me a filthy look and tease that I was that mean doctor who put that horrible tube in her chest.

One of the things that I have always loved about my job, and that transplants deliver in spades, is the opportunity to get to know people. Not just a superficial knowledge either:

transplants afford us the opportunity to have a longer, more in-depth relationship with these people.

For the better part of a year, I got to know Judy and her family so well. And for the better part of a year, Judy waited for the phone call that would change her life.

For most people who have an LVAD, the machine acts as a 'bridge to transplantation'. It keeps the patient alive, most importantly, but it also allows them to live their life relatively symptom-free from heart failure. Patients have travelled, danced, walked the City to Surf (an annual fun-run event in Sydney), gone to weddings or just gone to work. Of course, life is different, constantly attached to a machine. It's punctuated by medications and batteries and alarms—in the event of a power disconnection, the device alarms so aggressively your neighbours would be sure to hear it, for obvious reasons. But LVADs have been game-changers for people like Judy. What we really want, though, is that phone call that a heart has become available because then the patient can be free of the machine.

For the whole year that Judy was on her LVAD, every time I got a call about a transplant, if the blood type was the same, my thoughts immediately went to her. Could this be her heart? I wanted her to get a new heart so badly, and one night that call finally came. I took down the details of where I was going and when I'd be leaving. I listened to the details about the donor: their height, weight, how the heart was looking and their blood group. 'Who is the heart for?' I asked, silently praying it was going to be the answer

I wanted. 'It's for Judy,' came the answer, and with that tears rushed down my face.

In the middle of the night, my team and I made the journey to collect Judy's second chance at life. My heart was full the entire time. I was so thrilled to be a part of her journey from beginning to end—while at the same time wishing that we'd never had to meet. As she went off to sleep, placing all of her trust in the team, the theatre nurses told me she kept asking where I was. 'Nikki's gone off to get your heart,' they told her. Bringing that heart back for the implant surgical team will forever remain one of the highlights of my career. Judy was already asleep when I returned, the surgery underway, but as I dropped the heart off I peeked under the drapes, put my hand on her forehead and whispered, 'I'll see you soon, good luck,' despite knowing she couldn't hear me. I just wanted her to be okay, more than as a doctor. We all felt like a kind of strange extended family by now.

Just two days after the surgery, I heard that Judy was awake and so I raced into her room in ICU. I could feel happy tears pricking at my eyes as I stood at the door of her room, with her son and her husband. That room was so full of joy and happiness; it was the best place in the world at that very moment.

Judy wanted to listen to her new heart, so I got her a stethoscope and placed it in her ears, navigating my way around all of the lines and paraphernalia that she was still attached to. I held the stethoscope to her chest and she listened quietly before a smile crept across her face. 'That's my heartbeat,' she said and turned to her son. 'Mummy's got a heartbeat again.'

The tears weren't pricking at my eyes anymore; they were in full flow down my face.

I was a part of that. I was just one little part of a cast of many wonderful people—doctors, nurses, perfusionists, physiotherapists, exercise physiologists and many more—but, nonetheless, from the beginning to the end of her surgical story, I had been there. And it was and always will be one of the most memorable and uplifting times of my life. Not just because it was what we might call a 'great save', a life pulled from the brink when the odds were stacked against her. It was the human connection of this, the emotion, the joy, the fear, the hope, the love and the care. That equalled, maybe even outweighed, the medical miracle that had taken place over the course of the almost year and a half it had taken to get to this point.

Judy's husband caught that moment of listening to her heartbeat in a video on his phone, which he very kindly sent to me. I still have that video and I have watched it countless times. For all of the other things I love about medicine, like the intellectual challenge and the fascination with the human body, there is something truly special about human moments like this. And these moments are like *my* medicine: they're the perfect antidote to anything that is wrong or hard about this job.

8

CONSULTANT SURGEON
The downside

I started medical school when I was eighteen. Which meant, as a medical student in my late teens and early twenties, I was seeing things that many people had never experienced in their lifetimes. I still remember an elderly woman having a massive stroke and the emergency doctors telling her family she was unlikely to survive the night. I saw babies being born with terrible illnesses needing emergency surgery. It seemed so normal that it never struck me as horrendously unusual to be exposed to that much suffering so young.

I was in my fifth year of medical school when I was in the emergency department on an internal medicine rotation. The ED consultant came through the curtains that separated the resuscitation area from the rest of the department and hollered out for anyone who wanted to practise CPR to go behind the curtain with him. The resuscitation bays were five specially equipped bays for the sickest of patients who came through the ED—those in cardiac arrest, the people who had had terrible accidents, anyone whose life literally hung in the balance.

My registrar pushed me towards the consultant. 'You should go do some CPR,' she told me. I'd done CPR before; I'd even done it by the side of a road when I stopped at a car accident once. CPR always struck me as the pinnacle of trying to save someone's life, literally trying to squeeze their heart to keep life in the rest of their body by driving blood around when they can't.

CPR is a team sport. Unlike what you see in the movies, it can go on for a painfully long time. Hollywood would have you believe that you push on someone's chest for just a handful of times, rub paddles together and then shock them back to life. The reality is not this optimistic. First of all, if your heart stops (called a cardiac arrest) outside a hospital, only ten per cent of people survive. Secondly, not everyone gets a shock. Very few heart rhythms can be 'restarted' by delivering a shock called defibrillation. And, finally, CPR can go on for a very long time, even over an hour, while we try everything we can to restart someone's heart and make sure that they have been given absolutely every opportunity to survive.

On that day as a student in the ED I went behind the curtain into the resuscitation bays, where a small army of doctors and nurses was valiantly trying to save this man's life. As I listened to the chatter, it became evident why we were being ushered in to do CPR. This man was about to die; there was nothing else anyone could do for him. He had suffered a massive heart attack, and despite 50 minutes of work by the team his heart showed no signs of recovery and his other organs—his kidneys, his brain—had been taken down too. With no chance of recovery in sight, we were to try to learn something from this terrible event.

If you've never done CPR, you won't know the physical nature of it. We stand above the patient, using our entire body to push down on the centre of their chest, compressing the heart between the sternum and the spine to squeeze blood out. Every few minutes, the breathless and often sweaty person is relieved by someone new. When you get tired your compressions get bad, and when your compressions get bad you do your patient a disservice.

When my turn came to do the CPR, I stood on the little step next to the bed so I could be at the right height to be an effective compressor. I pressed all of my weight into his chest and, although I knew that this man was going to die— or perhaps more accurately was already dead—I had some little thread of hope that maybe under my hands he would survive. He would rally against the odds, against the body that was too sick to survive. I don't know if that was my naivety or my innate optimism.

The ED consultant who was leading the resuscitation effort asked the nurse who was recording every second of CPR, every drug given, every action taken, how long we had been going for.

'It's 63 minutes now.' My hands continued to go up and down on his chest.

The ED consultant spoke again, to everyone in the team. 'All right, is everyone happy we stop there? Anyone have any ideas, anything we haven't done?' I kept going amid a chorus of shaking heads and emphatic nos from around the bed. And with that, the ED consultant placed his hand on my shoulders and told me to stop. I did. I pulled my hands away and finally realised that, under my hands, this man had died.

I took a moment to survey the faces of the doctors and nurses in the team. Nobody cried, nobody looked sad; there was just a solemn mood as people started to pack up the equipment that they had tried to use to restart his heart. The defibrillator was wheeled away; the enormous number of syringes and drugs that had been given to him in vain were thrown away. Two nurses started to attend to his body with great care, covering him, cleaning him to make him look like he was in a peaceful slumber rather than having just endured a fatal heart attack and over an hour of CPR. It was respectful but everything that happened was like a well-oiled machine. For the first time, the strangeness of this struck me.

I turned my attention away from the activity and inward to myself, where I noticed a strange mix of adrenaline from the CPR efforts, sadness that someone had died and fascination with the stoicism that everyone just functioned with. Despite the fact that I was sad, sad that someone's father or husband or son had just died and fully aware of the enormity of that, I couldn't cry. I didn't want to.

Then something more profound hit me. He had died under my hands. I could split hairs here and say that, in reality, his organs had ceased to function well before I touched his chest. But I was the last person to do CPR on this person, the last to try to will life into him. It was a strange feeling, realising that for the rest of my career I would see people die. I would be at their side. I would be holding their hands or their organs when they passed away. Or, even worse, and this is a reality for all doctors, I could make a mistake, knowingly or unknowingly, and cause their death.

The ED consultant came up to me, and although I didn't know him at all he placed his hand on my shoulder as he stood in front of me. 'Do you need to talk about what just happened?' he asked, offering the opportunity for a debrief. Part of me wanted to, just to talk about how fucked up it was that someone had just died—because, let's be honest, while it is a common part of life in hospital and an inevitability for us all, it's still shocking and confronting. But I didn't. I wanted to be stoic like everyone else, pack up all of my emotions and questions and do what everyone else was doing: getting ready to help the next person who would need us.

I shook my head. 'No, I'm fine, thank you,' forcing a smile on my face and heading back to find the rest of my internal medicine team, going back to my normal day as if nothing had happened.

While this burying of our feelings has some necessity, it's also incredibly abnormal by societal standards. As my career went on, where I was constantly surrounded by life-and-death situations, responsible for pulling people back from the brink of death, the stakes would continue to climb.

Because when you're a heart surgeon, the chance that someone will die goes up. And the chance that you might directly have had something to do with that escalates with it.

* * *

One of the first things you learn to do when you're just starting out as a junior doctor in cardiothoracic surgery is to take vein to be used on the heart. No operation is a solo pursuit but heart surgery, more than many other surgeries, is truly a team sport, and that's just the surgical team. Usually, while the consultant opens the sternum and harvests the most important conduit, the internal mammary artery, which is tucked under the breastbone on each side of the chest, the more junior members of the team start taking out vein from the leg or, sometimes, the radial artery from the wrist.

The vein in the leg we use is called the saphenous vein. It runs from the ankle all the way up to the groin, picking up little tributaries along the way to return blood from your leg to the big veins in your pelvis and on to the heart. You would have seen it before: it's the vein that gets wild and dilated in varicose veins. Decades ago, when the forefathers of cardiac surgery were trying to work out how to fix the hearts of people with blockages in their coronary arteries, the saphenous vein was volunteered since it was plentiful and your leg can spare it. When it's removed, the myriad other veins in your leg take over.

I still vividly remember learning how to do this part of the operation as an RMO in cardiac surgery. I'd make a cut above the ankle and find the vein, which when it's healthy is a glistening silvery colour. Then you cut the skin above the vein all the way up to the leg; the more bypasses someone needs the higher you go, as you'll have to fetch more vein. This isn't the tricky part. The tricky part comes with ligating (tying off) every single side branch that the vein has. The saphenous vein can have dozens and dozens of branches, some barely a millimetre and so fragile that you're scared to look at them. But you have to tie a silk suture or use tiny stainless steel surgical clips to seal each and every tiny side branches, for the very obvious reason that, if they leak, the patient could very easily bleed to death.

Harvesting vein is a weirdly exciting experience, because it is basically like an entire operation in and of itself. You cut the skin, you do the surgery underneath, you sew the skin back up. Not just that, it feels like your first taste of significant responsibility for someone's life. After all, the tiny tube about to be transplanted from the leg winds up carrying blood to someone's heart, so you had better not fuck it up. Aside from being the reason that the patient could bleed to death if you make a mistake, your vein is going to help keep that person alive. It has to be beautifully harvested with the utmost care. Any inadvertent damage you cause to it could make it block off and leave your patient with the same problems they went through this huge operation to treat.

When you've taken the vein out of the leg, it goes up to the top of the table where the consultant surgeon is continuing with the rest of the operation. While that happened, I would diligently close the leg. Leg wounds can be difficult to heal because their blood supply isn't as good as in other parts of the body so, again, every care must be taken. This seemingly insignificant role in the team was where I learnt some of the most important lessons of being a surgeon.

Everything matters: every stitch, every cut, every tie. And patients will always comment on how well you close their wounds as, to them, an indicator of how well the rest of the operation went.

Before the vein goes into the heart, the surgeon checks it to make sure that it works and has no holes. A small metal tube called a cannula slides into the vein and the surgeon injects it with a saline solution. As a junior doctor, I would stop what I was doing in the leg, which was usually closing the skin by that stage, and just stare at the vein I had harvested, silently praying for approval.

Most of the time it came, usually in the form of a joke.

'Well done, you should submit this as a case report,' the professor used to tell me. Case forms are a type of medical publishing in prestigious journals to record and disseminate something truly remarkable happening. The same professor would chastise me by joking about watering cans and showers for the entire case if he found one hole that he had to fix. For all his faults, getting pissed off in theatre was not one of them.

Other consultants weren't so forgiving. One day, I was struggling with a particularly difficult vein. Just ten or so centimetres up the leg, the vein looked too small (which they can be from time to time) and I kept getting lost in the anatomy of this particular leg. I asked the boss for help and he turned to his right to look at the leg and immediately screamed, 'Well, this is a fucking dog's breakfast, isn't it. How many fucking times have I told you that you cannot fuck up the fucking vein!' before grabbing the scissors and forceps from my hands to fossick around in the leg for a good ten minutes before admitting defeat. (He used to swear as a form of punctuation and yell as a matter of course.)

Despite being yelled at and despite having a learning curve like anyone else, I was still pretty good at taking vein. I was pretty good at surgery, full stop, even then. I learnt the skills I needed to, I did them well and I understood the gravity of what I was doing. Which was good, because for my whole career I had never had a vein I had taken go on to cause catastrophic bleeding in someone's heart.

That isn't just because I was good at what I did. It was also because I worked in a team that was headed by someone, a consultant surgeon, with whom full and ultimate responsibility lay. Problem with the bypass machine, difficulty with the anaesthetic, shitty saphenous vein? At the end of the day, the consultant surgeon was the person who bore the bulk of responsibility for any and all bad outcomes in a case, even if they weren't the person who caused the issue (or fixed it, for that matter) or even if it was just bad luck.

Even though my early days of learning how to do this relatively simple skill of cardiac surgery was about me learning the mechanics and the importance of care with your work, what I didn't appreciate at the time was I was also learning the responsibility that you bear when you are the boss. While I was watching the boss test my vein to see if I had done a good job, what I was also seeing was the consultant doing a good job. I was watching the professor make jokes while he made sure that the patient was safe and that everything was in order.

When I started being the actual surgeon, the one doing the heart surgery side of things, and even more so as the consultant, the responsibility rose exponentially. I can still recall the first time as a fellow when the registrar handed me a vein that the professor would have described as a watering can. The patient that day was a Jehovah's Witness, meaning they would not accept a blood transfusion due to their religious beliefs, so I was feeling the extra pressure of not making a single mistake that could lose a single red cell. Of all the days to get a vein that was barely usable, taken without the due care it needed, this was not it. It was a harsh lesson to learn; in a case like that, when everything is even more stressful and difficult than usual, I shouldn't have had the junior do that important part of the surgery, I should have done it myself. It was a lesson in responsibility that I had learnt but forgotten to apply that day.

CASE 12

A nice set of grafts was how I'd describe this patient. He was here for elective heart surgery: coronary artery bypass grafting, to treat angina caused by narrowed coronary vessels. Angina is a little different from a heart attack. The damage in angina, rather than from the heart being starved of blood supply and precious oxygen that kills its muscle cells, isn't caused in the same way and the heart muscle cells don't die. Nonetheless, it can progress and can be debilitating to live with, limiting how these people live their lives as they try to avoid the painful and frightening attacks of angina.

This man was the sort of case we would joke was a 'gift'. A nice patient, a heart that was working well (even with the blockages), good targets (meaning his coronary arteries were nice and big without too many blockages that would make the operation technically difficult). In my notes before surgery, when I had met him in clinic, I had written 'excellent conduit, great targets', which meant this should be a slam dunk.

Operations like this are important from time to time. The cognitive load of emergencies and challenging cases, which in this hospital happened in the toxic environment of politics and under-resourcing, takes its toll. I didn't become a heart surgeon to do the easy cases or shy away from the difficult realities of life in a hospital but every now and again I welcomed a day like this, where the stress was lowered for once.

The music set the scene, my standard and, I hoped, uplifting and minimally offensive '80s and '90s tracks to which I would encourage the entire theatre to break into song. Helping me that day were two registrars, my more senior registrar and one of our more junior registrars. My senior registrar offended me by not recognising the Spice Girls. It was the sort of case where everything just went well, so well that I could tease him the entire time for not being aware of such a significant piece of pop culture.

As I opened the pericardium to expose the heart, I couldn't believe my luck. The heart was beating strongly and every coronary artery was perfect for grafting. My registrar, standing opposite me, repeated everyone's sentiment: 'This guy is such a gift, even I could do this!' And he absolutely could have, not just because everything was so straight-forward either. I almost felt guilty doing the case myself, but after a few weeks of dissections in the middle of the night and sick hearts hanging on for dear life, I needed the therapy of a case like this.

My junior registrar proudly handed me up the vein, and like I had seen my bosses do years before I gently inflated it and whistled under my mask, 'Very nice!'—a compli-ment to the patient and the budding surgeon alike. I quickly examined the entire length of vein and nothing caught my eye. We had done everything we needed to and I was ready to go.

With the conduits harvested and the heart on display, I could proceed with the real guts of the surgery, doing the grafts. I did the majority of my coronary artery bypass grafting (CABG, pronounced 'cabbage' for short) without a heart–lung bypass machine, called 'off-pump' or 'beating heart' surgery. Rather than having the machine take over the work of the heart and lungs, the heart keeps beating as we gently manipulate its position to do the bypasses and the lungs just carry on as normal. It's a labour-intensive way of doing the surgery for us all. For me, it's technically more challenging, using a completely different set of skills, even instruments. Every time I move the heart, the anaesthetist has to adjust medications and give fluid to support it as, funnily enough, the heart isn't a fan of being pushed around. Even the perfusionist, who would normally be running the heart–lung bypass machine, has to be at the ready in case something bad happens, which one perfusionist told me is harder than actually running the pump itself.

I started by grafting the most important vessel of the heart, the left anterior descending on the front of the heart, which supplies blood to the bulk of the all-important left ventricle. Off-pump surgery uses a special kind of retractor called a stabiliser that dampens down the rocking of the heart but doesn't eliminate it entirely, still leaving me to sew to a moving target. But since this case was a gift, it wasn't as hard as it had been in other people. I used a tiny scalpel blade to make a cut into the artery, just a few millimetres long. Since blood still flows through these vessels in off-pump surgery, I placed a tiny tube inside the vessel, called a shunt. Its job is to keep blood flowing to the heart beyond the cut I had just made and stop blood spraying all over the place.

With that in place, I could start sewing the internal mammary artery on. There are no machines for this, just me, my instruments and a piece of suture about the thickness of a hair. I had spent many hours practising this sewing, a join called an anastomosis. Each suture had to be perfect, just like the leg wounds I had sewn up all those years ago. One stitch slightly out of place and I could distort the entire join, impairing blood flow to the coronary artery, the exact opposite of what I was trying to achieve.

Once I had finished this, I repeated the process another three times to other coronary arteries around the heart. Open the vessel, place the shunt, sew it on a vein this time. With the last anastomosis done, I looked up at the clock. It was only 4.30 p.m., meaning that if everything continued to go well we could be out of there at a normal time. No midnight finishes for a change.

'Oooh!' I exclaimed. 'I might actually make it to the gym and be able to cook dinner!' and the theatre started to fill with the sounds of everyone planning out their own evenings. This is so uncommon, partly because finishing on time is not to be expected in cardiac surgery but also because we're superstitious and never tempt fate by planning for our lives outside the hospital.

My optimism was not misplaced; everything looked amazing at the end. There was no bleeding, the heart was happy, and with that, the skin was closed and the patient was being packed up to start his recovery in intensive care. And me, well, I was walking back to my car with a deep

sense of relief and satisfaction. Maybe I'm actually a pessi-
mist deep down, because when everything goes well I always
feel relief. Or maybe I just know too well how quickly things
can turn.

A few hours later, my phone rang. The intensive care
consultant's name flashed up on the screen, which is rarely a
good sign after 8 p.m.

'Nikki, your man from this afternoon has just dumped
three hundred into his drain,' referring to the man whose
operation had been about as textbook as it could possibly
have been. The intensivist told me that my registrar was
on the way in, and that, along with 300 millilitres of fresh
blood that had just poured into the drains I had left around
his heart to monitor for this exact issue, the patient's blood
pressure had started to drop.

I threw on some shoes and grabbed my keys to race out
the door. I lived about 20 minutes from the hospital but
I tempted fate and made it in just under 15 minutes, running
from the car park to the ICU. As the doors to the unit
swung open I saw the thing that I hate the most in the
world—a flurry of activity around the bed of my patient.
Pushing past the cast of thousands who had gathered—
some writing notes, others hanging bags of blood, some
just looking deeply concerned—I went straight to the chest
drains. Since I had left my house, another 800 millilitres had
dumped into the drain.

I hadn't been in the room even a minute before I announced
over the top of the hum of all the work going on, 'He needs

a take-back, now.' I hated take-backs. I would do just about anything to avoid them. A take-back meant that we were taking the patient back to theatre, usually because something like this massive bleeding had happened. I hated them with such passion because not only did it mean someone was sick but I also saw it as a deep failure of something I had done, or not done. I also especially hated doing them if it was after midnight and I was already asleep, because the only thing worse than being woken up was being woken up by what I would always think of as my own failure.

We got the patient back into theatre as quickly as possible, all the while the drains continuing to fill before our eyes. At the same time, his blood pressure became more and more precarious. Our team, so optimistic at their night off, had all regrouped once more but the joviality was long gone.

It takes less than a minute to get back into someone's chest after heart surgery. I ran a scalpel up the suture line that we had so carefully sewn not that long ago, and then quickly snipped each of the stainless steel wires holding the sternum together. As I pulled the sternum apart, blood and clots welled up around the heart and I was very aware of the anaesthetic team pumping in blood and medications to try to stabilise the blood pressure. Whatever was happening, it wasn't good. I sucked away the blood to try to see what had happened.

The blood kept coming, telling me that something was bleeding and it was bleeding a lot. When this happens, I need to check every hole I had made in the heart and I went systematically from the front to the back. As I lifted the heart, I saw the problem. The saphenous vein was hosing blood, by the looks of it from one of the tiny little side branches.

'Nikki, the pressure . . .' my anaesthetist said to me from over the drapes. I looked up. The blood pressure was barely recordable, a combination of massive blood loss and me lifting the heart. I placed a surgical sponge over the bleeding vein to try and settle some of the bleeding even just a little but the blood pressure was still hovering dangerously low. I had to make a decision right then and there: whether to chance it and wait for a perfusionist to get to the hospital so we could use the heart–lung bypass machine or whether I could fix it without it.

I would try to fix it now. I had no choice: he couldn't wait the half hour it would take for a heart–lung bypass machine.

I would use every trick I knew, every instrument, every stabiliser and the rest of the team would do the same. I knew this would be rough but I had to try to stop this bleeding and we would have to try to recover afterwards.

I tipped the heart out of the chest so I could see the bleeding aggressively beating out of the vein. I put my hand out to my scrub nurse for the suture and, without missing a beat, she placed it in my hands. I could feel myself holding my breath as I took the fine blue suture and placed a figure-of-eight stitch around the small hole that had caused so much trouble and then tied a knot as securely as I could without causing more damage, always a possibility in situations like this.

As the knot snugged down, the bleeding stopped but so did the blood pressure. I quickly released the heart back into the chest and placed my hand around it, squeezing the heart with internal cardiac compressions as the anaesthetic team poured in more blood and more fluids and every drug they could to bring the blood pressure up. I held my breath once more as I silently willed the ship to right itself. With the hole plugged we actually had a chance and, slowly but surely, the blood pressure rose. I watched the heart fill with blood rather than be dangerously empty.

I was there for another hour, triple checking every suture line, every side branch, every cut surface. I washed away the old blood and the anaesthetists corrected everything the massive blood loss had upset: they replaced the blood that had been lost, changed medications, gave others that would stop future bleeding and antibiotics to prevent infection. I looked up at the clock, which had just ticked past midnight, and sighed. Now that the adrenaline had slowed in my own body, I realised that I was tired and then a whole flood of thoughts started.

I was humiliated. I hate complications; I hate the idea that my mistakes could be responsible for someone's demise. And I hated the fact that everyone would be talking about this dramatic take-back at work tomorrow. Some would be sympathetic, proud of the way we managed it. Some would imply that I had done a really bad job, whether that was true or not.

I knew that walking into that ICU the next morning, I would feel immense shame at what had happened, especially knowing that this precarious situation could easily have had a terrible outcome. No matter how this had happened, the buck stops with me—I am responsible for everything that happens to that patient. The guilt of knowing something bad had occurred was like being kicked again and again.

The next day, the junior registrar came to find me. He looked about as guilty as I had felt the evening before, because he had taken the vein that had been the source of the troubles.

'Nikki, I heard what happened and I'm really sorry.'

I am not proud of the thought that popped into my head. Because the first thing I thought was that he should be. I was pissed off, not at him, just that we had experienced a complication. I was tired, grumpy and still carrying around a bit of shame and guilt.

'It happens, but now you've experienced this kind of thing, trust me, you won't do it again.'

It was meant to be reassuring but I don't know if it was. And although I was angry, it wasn't with my registrar. I was angry that I had needed a nice case and what I'd got instead was yet another sleepless night. I was angry that this complication had risked someone's life, and that his family had spent a sleepless night too, worrying about whether he was going to be okay. I was angry that a tiny part of me wanted to yell at everyone—at anyone—for this error and that those feelings would make me dangerously like the bosses who had screamed at me over the years, whom I desperately did not want to be like.

But mainly, I was angry with myself. I was furious that I had missed a tiny defect in the vein that had turned into a massive, life-threatening problem. But this was the cold, harsh reality of being a doctor and especially of being a heart surgeon.

You can cut to cure but you can just as easily do the exact opposite.

CRITICAL REFLECTION QUESTION
What do you observe about the life of a cardiothoracic consultant in this case study?

9

CONSULTANT SURGEON

No place for a bleeding heart

'Maybe we can have a quiet afternoon then?'

Every head in the cramped ward office snapped around at the RMO, who had just committed the cardinal sin of muttering what is referred to as the q-word. Half a dozen doctors and nurses looked as though they could have quite easily held him down and tortured him right then and there. I, for one, would have fully endorsed it. (Just to be clear, this is sarcasm and I would never actually endorse systematic torture of my junior staff. Even one who said the q-word.)

For a group of people who are so well versed in science, hospital staff observe far too many superstitions. We believe that a full moon will bring multiple patients to the ED with strange ailments and big personalities, a notion that has actually been scientifically disproved (yes, someone actually studied this). That certain weather conditions are associated with people with certain diseases coming to ED, even though there is absolutely no causative pathway whatsoever.

We believe that presentations of unusual or serious conditions always come in threes. In cardiac surgery, we're firm believers in the rule of threes. Transplants always come in threes, aortic dissections always come in threes. Basically, for any major emergency, expect three in a row.

And then there is the belief that some people are shit magnets—whenever they're at work or on call, it's guaranteed to be a busy day.

My most fervent superstition is that I have an unlucky scrub cap. Every time I've worn it (a grand total of three times), I've had a terrible day at work, which is clearly the fault of the scrub hat. Sadly, it's my Wonder Woman hat, which was a gift from one of my favourite scrub nurses. Now it sits at the bottom of my wardrobe where it can't cause any mischief.

By far and away the biggest superstition, though, that every single person who works in a hospital knows to pay extraordinary respect to, is the q-word. As a medical student, I remember walking into the ED with one of the more senior medical students. The department was uncharacteristically deserted. There were no beds in corridors, no patients overflowing from the cubicles and the perpetual noise of the department was conspicuously absent. I remarked, 'Wow, it looks quiet down here,' when the learned and wiser student turned around to me and hissed, 'Do not ever, *ever* say the q-word. Ever.' A sympathetic ED nurse, who heard the exchange, explained to me that urban legend has it that if it is q-word, and then you utter the q-word, all hell would break loose very soon afterwards.

No q-word. Got it.

It seems that this cardinal rule of hospital life had slipped the mind of my RMO that afternoon. My afternoon case had been cancelled because the hospital was bursting at the seams. Every patient who has cardiac surgery must go to the ICU afterwards, to be watched like a hawk and where high-level treatments like medicines to support the blood pressure and ventilation can be provided. When the hospital is overflowing, the ICU almost inevitably feels the brunt and any planned admissions (even cardiac surgery) to the ICU are postponed to leave room for unexpected admissions, like cardiac arrests from the ward patients or traffic accidents. My afternoon case was a very stable, elective case and, since there was no bed for her after her surgery in the ICU, she was put off until the following week. Which left a big gaping hole in my afternoon, an all-too-common occurrence with the ICU often full.

But my resident had just muttered the q-word. Obviously, I'm aware that whatever transpires afterwards is not *actually* his fault, but if you speak the q-word, you *will* be subjected to some good-natured teasing about whatever disaster you've manifested by tempting the fates or your deity of choice with your blatant disregard for the rules of hospital life. That afternoon, rather than operating, I'd decided to get a hot chocolate and do some teaching for the junior doctors.

(I hate coffee. Hate it. Don't @ me.) But no sooner did I have my hot drink in my hand that the afternoon took a drastically different direction.

CASE 13

My phone blared at me (my ringtone at the time was the first few bars of Nirvana's 'Smells Like Teen Spirit'—belligerent enough to ensure that when it rang it couldn't be ignored) and my registrar's name flashed up. 'What's up, mate?' I said to him, assuming he wanted me to grab him a coffee.

'Stamps, can you come down to ED? They've rung me about a stabbing.'

That was all he needed to say. I left my hot chocolate on the counter of the cafe and literally ran out, down the stairs to the ED two floors below, to find a cast of thousands milling around a resuscitation bay, preparing for the patient about to come in.

The emergency consultant found me. He was a tall, imposing man and an excellent doctor whom I'd worked with for many years now. There was no time for pleasantries and catch-ups today; he gave me the run-down of what they were expecting. The ambulance will call ahead on a dedicated phone line when they have a truly critical patient, giving vital details and an estimate of how far away they are to allow the ED to prepare. This call was a dramatic one—a 21-year-old man had been stabbed in the middle of the street in broad daylight during an argument with another young man. The paramedics had arrived to find the young man talking, but as they loaded him into the ambulance his heart stopped. They were moments away, doing lifesaving CPR. The ED doctor had rightly mobilised the entire hospital, including me and my team, for the possibility that he would need expeditious, lifesaving heart surgery.

I listened to the story and immediately decided what needed to be done: to save his life, I was going to have to open his chest right there in the emergency department. I sent my registrar to fetch the equipment in the ED and my surgical gloves and told him how he could assist me. The ED consultant wasn't so convinced. 'Are you sure? Don't we want to do an X-ray and an echo first? Or, why don't you put a chest drain on the left, I can do one on the right and we can see what happens from there?'

I looked him dead in the eyes. This was not the time for stuffing around; these situations needed decisive action, not tests that create inevitable and costly delays. 'Look, you can do whatever you like on the right side. The second he gets onto that bed,' I said, pointing at the resus bay bed, 'I'm opening his chest.' I'm not exactly known for being backwards in coming forwards at the best of times, but in an emergency I take charge probably more so than usual. (A man would be called assertive in this situation; the ED staff used to call me 'intense. Great, but intense.')

I could hear the paramedics coming down the corridor. Even in an emergency situation like this, the way in which the paramedics transfer the patient to the care of the ED is lyrical, a smooth process that is universally observed to ensure everyone knows what is going on with the patient. A nurse had taken over CPR from the paramedics, who were no doubt exhausted after doing CPR for the entirety of the eight-minute drive to us.

The paramedic began: 'I'll make this quick. This man was stabbed once in the chest. He had signs of life when we arrived but lost output in the ambulance. He has no access [referring to IV access to give drugs or fluids]. No known medical conditions. CPR duration about eight minutes.' And in the time that he spat out that information, the patient was on the resus bed and I was literally throwing Betadine onto the left side of his chest. No time for dainty painting here, just the need to get on with it.

An emergency room thoracotomy is the ultimate life-saving (and last-ditch) procedure. It's most often done when someone is stabbed in the chest and we need to access the heart to repair the hole that is killing the person, or relieve a condition called tamponade. A bleeding heart will gush into the pericardium, a rigid sac that the heart is contained by. It has no capacity to swell and so, as blood accumulates in the pericardium, it squashes the heart, suffocating it so it can't eject blood around the body. A thoracotomy describes an incision on the side of the chest that we can use to access the heart, the lungs or both.

There are a few other reasons we do this lifesaving procedure but, despite its heroic-sounding nature, it sadly doesn't save a life very often. Fewer than ten per cent of people survive it (this is a best-case estimate) and a paltry two per cent leave the hospital as they were beforehand; the patient's brain is often injured from even a brief period without blood supply.

The Betadine stained the skin of his left chest a deep brown, creating an illusion of sterility and bringing colour to his skin, which had turned greyish from no blood circulating. In reality, it feels like a token effort since the cleanliness of this procedure is not on par with the pristine cleanliness of a controlled operation in an operating theatre, but desperate times call for desperate measures. I shouted out for CPR to stop and everyone to step back, safely removed from the chaos of sharp instruments flying rapidly.

I took my scalpel and made an incision in a line that curved just under the left nipple, extending from the side of the breastbone right around into the armpit, as far back as I could possibly go. The blade passed through the skin and the subcutaneous fat, and scraped over the top of the intercostal muscles, the thin muscles between the ribs that aid breathing. I relinquished my scalpel for a big pair of scissors and plunged them between the ribs, opening the blades and stripping the muscles off the ribs, allowing me inside the chest. I thrust the left lung out of the way to show me the pericardium, which I could see was bulging and full of blood. I took my scissors again and stripped open the pericardium to deliver the heart out of its home. The blood that was strangling the heart spilled out into the left chest.

I had no concept of how long it had taken me. But my other registrar did. 'It took you 30 seconds, a minute tops:

I watched,' she told me later. In less than a minute (apparently), I had this man's broken heart in my hand. Immediately, I could see the problem staring back at me, a small wound to the right ventricle. '4-0 prolene, double-loaded!' I yelled. My registrar thrust into my hand the needle holder we had already prepared, loaded with the suture, a little finer than fishing line, which I plunged into the heart around the hole the knife had left, sealing it closed. I squeezed the heart in my hands. It was empty; most of his blood volume had spilled out. His heart quivered; it didn't beat in the rhythm it needed to. I tried to force life back into it and blood around the body.

'Get access in the leg!' I directed my registrar to cut down onto a large vein in the leg to directly deliver lifesaving blood and fluids. The patient's circulation was collapsed; everyone was struggling to access his veins. I had plugged the hole in the bucket but the bucket was empty. 'Give me an adrenaline syringe!' I shouted out to whoever could give it to me. One of the ED nurses passed me the syringe and needle, which I shoved directly into his heart. As I pushed down on the plunger, my registrar had gotten into a vein and started to squeeze in fluids. I kept squeezing on the patient's heart and, all of a sudden, the adrenaline and the blood transfusion kicked in and the heart sprang to life. This is why I love the heart. You can stab it, empty it, hold it in your hands and it can still recover. How something can be so delicate yet so resilient is poetry to me.

As the young man's heart started beating again, his blood pressure started to climb. I looked around me, finally having a moment to take in what else was going on rather than my absolute focus on the heart. The room was full, many watching the drama unfold and many working tirelessly to save a life. My anaesthetist and her registrar were placing a central line in his neck to give more blood and medications. We had secured the drip in the cut my registrar had made in the leg. The ED doctors and nurses were placing monitoring and drawing up drugs out of shiny glass vials, and the orderlies were running in and out, absolutely vital in delivering the blood that desperately needed to be replaced. The teamwork was phenomenal and I'm glad that I took that second to look around and appreciate it.

Stability was finally achieved; the young man's heart was beating strongly. As I placed my hand around his heart I could feel that it was once again full, that we had finally replaced much of the blood that had been lost. At this stage, we needed to move out of the ED and into the operating theatre, to clean the chest and close it up carefully. The operating theatres were on the floor above the ED at the other side of the hospital—a legacy of renovations and departmental moves over many years—and I can tell you that careening through a hospital corridor and then taking an elevator ride with a patient whose heart had been flaccid and inactive just minutes earlier seemed precarious. Nobody wants to manage a cardiac arrest inside a moving tin can if they can at all help it.

As we bundled through the doors of the operating theatre complex, safely out of the elevator, I could hear one of the theatre nurse managers shouting that we couldn't go into theatre as the case wasn't booked on the computer system. What would she have me do: wait in the corridor until the paperwork was done?

Every case had to be booked into a kind of online diary that the nurse managers of the theatre would use to coordinate the operating theatres and the staff for those operations. It's obviously a necessary process to run a smooth department, but the phone call we had given them to tell them we had to come up in a hurry apparently didn't suffice, even at a time like this.

This is hospital bureaucracy; not even having your left lung and heart on display, with me elbow deep in the chest, will allow for an exception to the system, or for one of the managers to help us out and do the inane online form for us. Lifesaving after paperwork, please. I told my team to keep moving to theatre anyway because there was no way in hell I was stopping for paperwork. I got a written complaint for violating protocol and had to explain my actions a few weeks later, which involved me exercising an enormous amount of self-control not to tell the bureaucrats to go to hell.

In the operating theatre, I carefully closed every opening I had made, erasing the evidence of the invasive and aggressive incursion into the young man's chest. By some miracle, his heart was unwavering, steadily beating away as though it had never been violated. First by a knife, during an argument gone very wrong, and then by me, grabbing it from its cocoon to sew it closed. Eventually, the patient was safely moved to the

ICU and kept asleep with a breathing tube connecting him to a ventilator, while we waited to see if he would remain stable and, more importantly, if his brain had survived undamaged.

CRITICAL REFLECTION QUESTION
What do you observe about the life of a cardiothoracic surgeon in this case study?

In the next few days, there were emails to everyone involved. One from me, many from the ED, all congratulating everyone involved on a truly outstanding team effort. And it was. Although it seems like a heroic effort from one person, every single person involved was a hero. These situations only succeed because of the efforts of many. We were right to congratulate each other and to share in the modicum of success we had achieved because, as I've already said, the wins in these kinds of situations are few and far between.

Sadly, though, our win was to be short-lived. In the ICU, the medications that were keeping our man asleep were slowly wound back. It's the only way to make an initial assessment of what the brain is doing. In the fog of sedatives that keep people asleep (so that we can safely care for every organ system), the brain's abilities are lost. As the sedation wore off, it became clear that the patient's brain had suffered irreparable damage. A CT scan of his brain confirmed the extent of the damage. Despite the outstanding treatment from the paramedics onwards, we hadn't been able to save his brain from catastrophic damage. After telling the family of this devastating finding, his life-support machines were turned off and death finally took him.

***

'The adrenaline rush doesn't last forever,' my boss warned me.

It was a Friday night and we were taking an emergency to theatre, an aortic dissection. I was a junior doctor, just an RMO in the unit, and I was absolutely enamoured with cardiac surgery. I especially loved the emergencies, the opportunities for dramatic saves, the chance to alter the course of a life-threatening illness.

Whenever something like that happened, I could feel the adrenaline coursing through me. I loved emergencies, even as a medical student. The pressure never scared me; instead I tended to thrive in those situations. I could think quickly and act just as fast, and I trusted myself and my team to rise to the occasion. And what better way to apply your hard-earned skills and knowledge than by stepping up to the plate when it mattered most?

I used to worry that there was something wrong with me to be getting so excited by such traumatic occurrences in someone else's life. Like I was somehow getting a thrill from suffering. One Saturday, I was at work (as per usual) in the afternoon, ready to start a heart transplant. I ran into a friend who was a doctor in the ICU and told her excitedly that we were doing a heart transplant shortly.

I was genuinely excited. I loved transplant surgery and I had gotten to know the recipient well over the preceding months. He was basically just a kid who was about to get a chance at life after spending six months attached to his LVAD, a mechanical heart that let him go back to school while he awaited the life-changing phone call.

I was so thrilled to be a part of it, so jumped up on adrenaline and hope that I forgot for a second that not everyone in the ICU was having as good a day. In a room near where I stood with my friend, an equally young man lay dying, his family wrestling with the fact that, after a car accident, their son might never wake up. I hated myself in that moment for being so gleeful.

But the adrenaline rush, the excitement to do the very thing I wanted to do, mattered so much to me. On that Friday night when other people my age were at the pub, my idea of a great night was to spend six or seven hours scrubbed at an operating table. The juxtaposition of me nearly jumping around with excitement and my boss being openly annoyed at the same time prompted him to try to warn me that my youthful exuberance would fade.

Defiant, I told him that there was no way I would ever stop loving this. I just couldn't fathom how the elation I got with everything we did could ever vanish. Some of this was simply me being naive. I hadn't had twenty years of being woken up at three o'clock in the morning, of missing kids' birthdays and a divorce to tarnish my love of fixing people's hearts.

I was still deeply and desperately in love with this job. This job, which I put above and beyond all else, made me feel alive. Whether it was those emergencies or the planned operations that were decidedly less dramatic, I loved every moment of it. That adrenaline rush, that moment when you could reach into someone's chest, literally hold their broken heart in your hands and then put it back together.

I was utterly determined to hold on to that awe and that love of what I did. If you didn't love it—and I mean truly and deeply love what you did—how were you going to get out of bed in the middle of the night to save someone's life? How would you take the care you need to in every cut, every suture? The way I saw it is that you couldn't possibly.

I once worked with a senior surgeon who could barely disguise his disdain for his job anymore. Emergencies made him fly into a rage, or attempt to rationalise why they didn't need to be emergencies, why they could wait until the morning. His prickly demeanour was the stuff of legend, as he constantly argued with his colleagues. He treated the system with contempt, and although the broken and inefficient healthcare system was certainly frustrating, his attitude wasn't something any of us ever wanted to emulate.

He completely lacked the love of what he did. The way he talked about his junior days, I always got the impression he used to have that same sense of awe and interest we all had. The fascination with how the heart worked and how we could fix it. The satisfaction of a job well done. But he had been so ground down by years and years of it that the sheen had most definitely worn off. When I heard that he had retired, I hoped that he had found something he loved to dilute the cynicism that had brewed over the years.

On the day that young man was stabbed, I could feel the adrenaline. I still felt as I had since I was a junior doctor: the prospect of saving someone's life; the awe, as I looked up and saw a team of dozens of people—doctors, nurses, order-lies—all pulling together, doing their best work and using all of their skills to try to save that young man's life.

He died, but not because we didn't try. We gave abso-lutely everything and then some to save his life. And when we realised that he would never wake up, it hurt. The disap-pointment that our absolute best wasn't good enough is such a painful realisation. To realise that someone's brother, some-one's son, had died is a sobering moment, yet it was not going to erode my love for what I do. It was not what was going to transform me from that young doctor who wanted to change the world into something I wasn't sure I wanted to be.

I remember once being told that operating is the easy part of being a surgeon. You're so well trained in that for so many years, you can sometimes almost quite literally do it in your sleep. Even losing a patient, while incredibly hard, is some-thing we are taught to understand is a reality of what we do and to take steps to prevent that from happening wherever we can. The hard part of being a doctor, of being a surgeon, is everything else.

Around when that young man was stabbed, I started to notice something in myself. I still loved my actual job: that is, operating. But I was finding myself getting increasingly down about everything else I had to deal with. It was starting to tarnish my love for being a surgeon as I'd sworn it never would, and that scared me more than having to perform emergency surgery in the middle of an ED ever could.

Something had started to happen that shocked me: I had started to dread coming to work. The operating theatre largely remained my sanctuary, but as I pulled into the car park each day, my thoughts almost immediately turned to all of the other things that would colour my day: whether I was going to have to fight for an ICU bed for my patient; the constant bickering between colleagues that I may or may not be involved in; endless bureaucratic emails that took up far too much time. Was this the stuff that would take the adrenaline rush away?

I decided to speak to someone about what I felt. Maybe just getting it all off my chest would make me feel better. It could even allow me to talk to someone with more experience and find a way to fix some of these problems that were getting me down. I decided to have dinner with one of my old bosses, the same guy who told me that the adrenaline rush wore off.

We met at a local pub for a meal one Saturday evening. As I arrived, he gave me a big hug and told me he'd always wanted a date with a blonde who wasn't his wife. I laughed uncomfortably, having listened to him make these kinds of jokes about all the blondes he'd worked with, and sat down and ordered a drink.

As I sipped on my wine, I told him 'I need this drink' and started to tell him what was wrong. I detailed how every day I turned up to work there was always something and it was getting me down. It was the cancellation of operations that meant you had to explain to a patient that they weren't getting their surgery. It was the bickering and political manoeuvring that seemed to be par for the course among my colleagues. I was just plain tired.

In exasperation, I threw my hands up in the air and said, 'Maybe I should just stop caring so fucking much.'

He grabbed my hands and smiled. 'Exactly.'

Many years ago, I'd promised myself that the day I stopped caring, or stopped loving this job, it would be time to go. Given that it takes so much of you, in my mind an undying love of this job was a prerequisite. You can't get out of bed at three a.m. for a job you only had lukewarm feelings for. You can't stand up for hours and hours on end if all you can think about was being somewhere else. You certainly couldn't prioritise the patient when you just didn't care.

My arrogance as a junior doctor, thinking that this would never happen to me, wasn't exactly misplaced. Even on days when I was being absolutely beaten down by the system I could still find solace in the cool, controlled room of an operating theatre, where it was just me, my team and the heart. I couldn't fathom ever falling out of love with that because it had never stopped being amazing to me.

Losing patients is traumatic, especially when they are young and you have pulled out all the stops. But by far and away the most traumatic thing about surgery is everything that isn't surgery. That's what wears you down, year after year. That's what robs you of the adrenaline rush at the thought of helping someone and your zest for jumping out of bed every single day. While nearly two decades of medicine had taught me what I needed to know about being a surgeon—the art and science of what I do and the resilience in the face of loss—there was something missing.

Surgery is wonderful but it is hard. It is hard enough without the perpetual pressure from bureaucracy and office politics. I wondered, how long can you hang on to that love to guide you through the obstacles of everything else? And how long can that love endure?

PART II
Scrubbed out

10

CHRISTMAS
The heart of the matter

As strange as it sounds, I actually enjoy Christmas Day ward rounds. Everyone greets each other with goodwill and a 'Merry Christmas'; the wards are decorated with creative Christmas decorations, featuring what would usually be hospital rubbish repurposed to make Christmas trees and garlands. Fairy lights are hung from every ward and virtually every staff member wears Christmas scrubs or Santa hats. Given that we were all there away from our families and friends, the atmosphere is unmistakably jovial.

As a junior consultant and a childless one at that, I had worked more holidays than not in the last ten years of my career. Which meant that I had accumulated a collection of Santa hats and reindeer antlers for the express purpose of a ward round, to add to the festive spirit.

I joined my registrar—also childless and junior relative to her colleagues—on our fantastical, reindeer-antler-wearing ward round through the hospital. The patients always made the best of the day, with their families bringing in gifts, children showing their parents or grandparents who were convalescing in uncharacteristically bright and cheery wards what Santa had brought them in the still of the night. If I could sum up Christmas Day in a hospital, it was everyone making the best of a sometimes bad situation.

This Christmas, not many people had it as bad as Michelle. Michelle wasn't my patient but she had undergone a brutal nine-hour surgery the day before by one of my colleagues. I'd popped in and out of her surgery because it was such a big one that, happily, I probably wouldn't see again for many years to come.

Michelle had been born with an abnormal aortic valve. The aortic valve's job is to keep blood from going backwards into the heart as it journeys around the aorta to our body, and it normally has three paper-thin leaflets that float in and out against one another, looking similar to an inverted parachute. Michelle's valve only had two leaflets, predisposing it to calcify and stiffen. If it was a parachute, Michelle's valve was like a badly packed one. As a result of this abnormality, Michelle's aorta had dilated to a dangerous degree. Like a balloon that's overfilled, Michelle's bloated and thin-walled aorta was at risk of rupturing and so, three years earlier, she had undergone surgery in another state to replace the valve and the first ten centimetres of her aorta.

Two weeks before Christmas, when she should have been shopping for gifts and planning her day with family, Michelle felt like someone had stabbed her in the chest. Her hands immediately went for the pale scar that adorned the middle of her chest as she alerted her husband that something was wrong. She was correct; somehow, bacteria had entered Michelle's bloodstream and travelled to her new aorta and aortic valve, where they had been slowly eroding the delicate joins between the prosthetic material and her own heart. Tiny amounts of blood were following the path set by the invaders and trying to burst free, creating a false aneurysm. A false aneurysm is basically a blood-filled sac that could burst; in Michelle's case, if it did she wouldn't survive.

I remember seeing Michelle's CT scans when she was first admitted and I can also remember feeling my own heart skip a beat. It was bad; the false aneurysm was sizeable, enough to warrant surgery. For two weeks, she stayed in hospital as the whole team tried to plan the best way to tackle this life-threatening problem. Picking the brains of the best doctors in the hospital, we ran through every possible solution but, in the end, the only way to fix the problem and protect Michelle was to perform risky surgery to re-replace her aortic valve and her aorta.

On Christmas Eve, Michelle hugged her children and gave her husband a kiss through a brave face, telling them that she'd see them on Christmas Day. Michelle's surgery was a marathon; everything was distorted and damaged by the infection even more than we'd expected. Repeat or, as we call it, re-do heart surgery is not for the faint-hearted. When you cut yourself on the skin, your body forms a scar. And when you do surgery on the heart that same kind of scar forms around it, encasing it, oftentimes making it challenging to get back into the chest.

For nine long hours my colleague, Michelle's surgeon, carefully chipped away at the scar tissue and removed the infection, connecting everything back together. I watched intermittently during the day between clinics and consults, and I can say without a doubt that it was one of the most challenging surgeries I'd seen. The long surgery had placed an extraordinary amount of strain on Michelle's heart and, in fact, on her whole body. My colleague rang me that night to hand over, since I was on call the next day; Michelle was on industrial doses of medicines to keep her heart pumping strong and rescue her blood pressure from dangerously low levels. 'We just need to hope she doesn't bleed overnight,' he said, since major bleeding after surgery is just another stress her body didn't need.

Michelle survived the night, still on an enormous amount of medicine to support her frail physiology. I went into her room in ICU, leaving my reindeer antlers at the door. It didn't seem like the time or place for frivolity or to remind Michelle's husband that his wife was in ICU after major surgery on a day they should be enjoying their family. As I stood by her bed, listening to the nurse and doctor from ICU fill me in on what had been happening overnight, my eyes wandered to the wall on Michelle's left.

Even in the short few hours she had been in ICU, the wall had been filled with pictures. Michelle, smiling at the camera. Her kids, toothless grins and school uniforms, placed as if they were watching over their mother. Even the family dog got a place on the wall, right next to Michelle and her husband on their wedding day. Michelle was my age, our birthdays separated by just a few short weeks. As that realisation dawned on me, I felt a pain in my soul. Life was, quite simply, unfair.

Despite everything, Michelle was hanging in there.

The registrar and I finished the ward round and I decided to do just a little paperwork at my desk. My own desk had no photos: no family, no kids, not even my poor cats had won a position next to my computer (terrible cat mother, I must be). Just thank you cards from patients and printed-out protocols provided a backdrop to a 3D model of a heart. The contrast was stark and my mind wandered to the differences between Michelle's life and mine.

My daydreaming was interrupted as my registrar flung open the door and said, 'ICU just rang; Michelle isn't looking well,' in breathless tones that let me know she had raced down the corridor to tell me. I hurried with her to the ICU, and as I walked in the door I could hear the piercing tones of the arrest bell.

Michelle was grey and the lines on the monitor showed that her heart had stopped. We had drilled this scenario dozens of times: if someone who has recently had heart surgery has a cardiac arrest, we open their chest in ICU.

The ICU nurses wheeled in the trolley of surgical instruments I needed to get into Michelle's chest to try to save her. It was a flurry of activity: antiseptic on the chest, drapes over her body, scalpel sliced through the recently placed sutures. I snipped the four stainless steel wires holding her breastbone back together and they pinged apart, splaying the sternum open.

Michelle's heart was eerily still. I cradled it in my right hand and squeezed, rhythmically. It wasn't until then that I looked up and watched the rest of the team working, hanging bags of fluid and blood, pushing medications through her intravenous lines. Squeeze, squeeze, squeeze. 'Come on, Michelle,' I thought as I looked at her smiling face and her family in the photos on the wall. Her heart lay still and in my hands it felt like stone. I ran through every possible scenario in my head as to why this had happened. It wasn't bleeding; it wasn't an abnormality in her electrolytes. Had something happened to the new valve? Unlikely, I thought. The only conclusion I came to was that Michelle's heart was broken. Broken by the infection that had ravaged it for weeks and too sick to handle the marathon surgery.

I decided to take Michelle from the improvised operating theatre I had turned her room into in the ICU across the corridor to the operating theatre. In the short trip, my hand didn't leave Michelle's heart as I kept squeezing it, trying to keep blood going to her vital organs, especially her brain.

Michelle's heart showed no signs of recovery; the only way to save her life was to put her on ECMO, to let the machine take over the work of her sick heart and, I hoped, let it recover. As the machine took over, I could feel tears threatening to spill out of my eyes into my mask. Michelle was safe, for now.

'Nikki, are these your reindeer antlers?' my registrar asked as we left ICU once Michelle was safe.

'Don't worry about them; chuck them out.' I didn't feel like wearing anything festive anymore. I felt defeated.

Two days later, Michelle died. Her heart made signs of recovery, but one morning the ICU nurses noticed that Michelle's left pupil wasn't constricting when the nurse shone light in it, a warning sign that Michelle's brain was sick, potentially catastrophically so. Connected to every machine known to humanity to keep as many organs alive as possible, Michelle went to the CT scanner, which revealed the tragic news that Michelle's brain had been irretrievably damaged.

When Michelle's heart had stopped, her brain had stopped getting blood. Virtually half of her brain was infarcted, meaning that her brain was actually dying. It was irreversible and irretrievable. For all intents and purposes Michelle's brain was dead, meaning that so was she. I sat silently in the family meeting with her husband and her mother, whom I had never met but whose faces were burned into my mind from their photos on her wall. I listened as the ICU doctor explained everything with such amazing compassion and offered a very simple and woefully inadequate, 'I am so, so sorry. We have done absolutely everything that we could for her.' Like that was supposed to put everything to rest.

My on-call finished that night; someone else was at the helm, which meant only one thing. Whisky. I sat on my balcony at home, trying to replay over and over in my head what I should have done differently, what we all should have done differently for Michelle. It wasn't the heart surgery that I couldn't get out of my head. It was those photos.

Michelle was my age. While I was sitting there, enjoying a whisky on my balcony, her family were no doubt in the greatest pain of their lives. Every Christmas, her daughters would be painfully reminded how on this day, however many years ago, their mother's heart stopped and never really started again. I pictured an ICU nurse handing her husband every photo that adorned that wall, knowing they would never see that smile again. But also that they would be proud of her and love her and carry her around forever.

My age. She was my age.

I'd always known I'd given up time with my family to be a surgeon, but that Christmas Michelle had made me wonder if I'd given up more than I'd realised.

***

When I was a medical student, the first time I went to theatre was so exciting. I was finally getting to wear scrubs, like a real doctor. It felt like a coming-of-age moment, stepping out of my child-like phase as a medical student and edging one tiny step closer to becoming a fully fledged surgeon.

In the female change-rooms, there was a large trolley

stacked with scrubs of two varieties. One side had what we liked to call 'boilersuits'—overalls that were white and threadbare, rendering them virtually see through and not at all cut to fit women. Nothing in surgery is made to fit women: the gloves fit poorly, the operating tables don't go low enough and the instruments are too big for our hands. Even the lead gowns we wear when using X-rays in an operation, meant to protect us from years of radiation, fit so poorly sometimes that they expose us in a way that can compromise our health. When I put the ill-fitting scrubs in that context, I feel bad for complaining that they're unflattering when they could be straight-out dangerous.

The alternative to the threadbare boilersuit was pants and a top, in a light baby blue. Given that their structural integrity was superior to the boilersuit (they weren't see through) and you could mix and match sizes to get something that vaguely fitted, they seemed a safer option. On my very first foray into the operating theatre, I made what I thought was the sensible decision to go with the baby blue.

Walking out of the change-rooms was kind of transformative, like Clark Kent had changed into his superhero lycra, and that was exactly what I felt like. I had, I thought, transformed into someone who looked like an actual surgeon. As I stepped through the doors to the theatres, my registrar looked at me and laughed, saying, 'Why are you wearing the nurse scrubs?'

I had had no idea there were nurse scrubs and doctor scrubs: why aren't they just scrubs? Would I have looked more like a doctor if I'd gone for the transparent white boilersuit that all the men wore, so transparent that it left absolutely nothing to the imagination? As it turned out, given that the vast majority of the female staff at the time who worked in the operating theatres were nurses and that the baby blue top and bottom set fitted women better than the boilersuits and gave some semblance of privacy, nurses predominantly wore the baby blues; they were hence called nursing scrubs. In my naivety, I couldn't comprehend how clothes could be gendered when these particular clothes sought to make us all the same, uniformed and alike. Every time after that, I carefully selected my underwear and sucked it up and wore the boilersuits, determined to prove that scrubs are not gendered but wanting to dress like a man—that is, a surgeon—all the same.

While the division between nurse scrubs and doctor scrubs seems ridiculous enough, some hospitals still stock scrub dresses, a throwback to the Florence Nightingale days of crisp white dresses. Why they still existed was beyond me: scrubs are surprisingly uncomfortable as it is, and doing CPR in a scrub dress is nothing short of ridiculous. In yet another way in which women can be ridiculed when working in health care, if you're wearing a scrub dress you are required to wear tights, lest you start a plague with something called 'pubic shed'. Which is yet another way for miserly old matrons to embarrass you for a phenomenon that doesn't exist and further make women in an operating theatre feel especially unwelcome.

Back at medical school, bright-eyed and innocent, my friends and I used to see the one or two consultant female surgeons in the change-rooms or the corridors of the operating theatre and whisper excitedly as they bustled past. It was like we had seen a celebrity and we would look at them with such admiration, just grateful to have been in their orbit if only for a split second. The most important feature of one of those women, though, was not the fact that she was world renowned in her field nor that she had led surgical teams through major disasters and saved countless lives with her research, but that she had done that *and* been a mother. She was held up as a beacon of how you can be both a surgeon and a 'real' woman.

When I used to talk about being a surgeon, one of the most common questions I was met with was 'How are you going to have children?', a question that made me cringe. How could perfect strangers ask me about one of the most personal aspects of my life? I hadn't even decided what I wanted; as a young woman, career obsessed in her early twenties, children seemed a world away. The conversation embarrassed me as I watched their reactions when I shrugged my shoulders and said that I didn't know. My only way of dealing with it became to make jokes to deflect the situation. 'It's okay, I handed in my ovaries when I started medical school,' I'd say, the laughter at my dry humour drawing their attention away from the most personal part of who I am long enough for me to change the topic.

As the years ticked by, the question became much less inquisitive and much more judgemental, peppered with warnings against winding up like an older female surgeon who was 'barren and alone' with nothing but her career and her dogs to keep her company. Those giving the advice always seemed to serve up an ultimatum: have children and you can't be a surgeon, or at least not a good one. Don't have children and be a cold-hearted bitch who is career obsessed. Nobody once stopped to ask me, if I did want to have a family, how they could make it easier for me, how they could help me achieve everything I wanted.

Nobody ever asked the men how they were going to balance children and their career. I've watched women in surgery, their pregnant figures squeezed into scrubs that were made for men, barely fit women and definitely didn't give a shit if you were growing a baby, endure accusations that they cannot possibly be committed enough to surgery if they were stupid enough to get knocked up.

As a student, women were absent. As an actual surgeon, we haven't come nearly as far as we should.

In Australia, just over twelve per cent of surgeons are women (this figure is comparable to other countries like the USA, UK and Canada). Let me give you some context to that. For several decades now, at least half of medical school graduates are female. So, if we were to think that once we had more female doctors things would equal out we'd be mistaken. There's not just a lack of female surgeons; a perpetually growing body of research into women in surgery and women in medicine has found that, when it comes to their careers, women get a rough deal. They're paid less, promoted less, harassed more and are more likely to leave surgery. In the workplace, they're treated worse by other staff members than their male counterparts. But it's okay. We can offset that by baking cookies, according to one research paper published in the prestigious *Journal of the American Medical Association* in 2020. In fact, I was once given that advice by a colleague who told me it was good that I baked for the team, 'otherwise people will definitely think you're a bitch'.

In Perth, my hometown, where I went to medical school and spent most of my career, if you have surgery the chances are you're getting a man. I was the only female cardiothoracic surgeon in that town for years. In fact, five surgical specialties had three or fewer female surgeons. What if you wanted a woman surgeon because you connected with her or felt safer with her? What if you wanted to be a surgeon, and everywhere you looked for a mentor all you saw was men who couldn't guide you through the unique aspects of juggling motherhood and a surgical career? Or what happens if you were doubling over with period pain but still had a full surgical list? Or just wanted to have someone who looks a little like you, whom you could relate to, just in arm's reach?

In recent years, we keep telling women that they can be whatever they want to be but, really, can they? We tell them that they can be great and that they belong in surgery, they just have to want it badly enough and be willing to rise above the slings and arrows. They have to prove themselves and earn their respect but so many of our male colleagues are assumed to be competent and receive deference by default. The only way to be accepted and to be successful is to be perfect, an unattainable combination of technically perfect, feminine and caring yet confident and assertive. But not too assertive or confident, lest you be called arrogant and be knocked down a peg or two. Sometimes, it's like we're martyring ourselves trying to achieve the impossible.

In my career, I plunged myself into improving the status of women in medicine and surgery by doing research or delivering keynote addresses at surgical conferences around the world. I even went to local schools to show the kids that surgery was an amazing career, to pay particular attention to the girls in the class and tell them that science was cool and never let anyone tell them that girls can't do something. My heart was so full as spreading this message seemed to be making a difference to these young minds. One Book Week little girls dressed up as me, because when they grew up they wanted to be surgeons too. But had we really changed the world or had I misled them all?

One of the recent talks on women in surgery I gave was at a surgical conference. It was an invited keynote presentation to make up for the fact that fewer than ten per cent of presenters at the conference were female and the organisers were publicly called out for that fact. I'm never a nervous speaker; in fact, I would rather talk to a full auditorium than have a one-on-one conversation. But that day, I was utterly petrified. Rather than give my keynote in the large main auditorium, I'd been sent to deliver my work in a small auditorium where I was so close to everyone I could probably read what they were watching on their phones rather than listening to the speaker. The hardest part was that some of the anecdotes or examples I had to share were about people who may have been sitting in that very audience.

For the first time that I could remember while giving a presentation, my voice shook as I described the objective data that showed how gender disparity in surgery impacts women both inside and outside a hospital's walls. The pay gap, the lack of promotion, the preponderance for women to leave surgery and the sexual harassment. And while I tried to find the courage to confront the very people who had been a party to these kinds of things, I watched heads in the audience shake in disbelief. Did I get through to anyone?

After my talk, I was sitting down outside the auditorium to chat to some colleagues I hadn't seen in a long time when I was interrupted by another colleague. We'd never worked together—I had met him once before—but he came up to me, hugged me and kissed me on the cheek. And as he chatted to me, he kept putting his hand on my leg and telling me how we needed to catch up before the conference ended. I wanted to either disappear into the chair or scream at him to keep his hands to himself. What a weak woman I was, just standing up on stage talking about how behaviours exactly like this had no place in our profession and, even as a consultant, when it happened to me I froze because I was too scared of making a scene and upsetting a man whom one day I might rely on to give me a job.

One of my few female colleagues found me afterwards and told me that maybe I needed to reconsider this push. 'Gently, gently,' she said. 'We need to make sure we don't upset anyone. Like you, I heard you bake for everyone at work.' It was true, I love baking for my team—brownies, cookies, cupcakes, anything to make the day pass a little more easily and to give a tiny token of my appreciation for what everyone does every day. Even as a surgeon, my ability to be maternal and nurturing to my team was as big a factor as whether or not I'm good at my job.

It seemed word of my speech had made it from the interstate conference back home when one of the other surgeons was caught telling a registrar how my take on things was very wrong. 'Dr Stamp thinks everything is about gender and it's not. It's mostly in her head. These young women would be better off following the advice of someone else. She's just a crazy feminist.'

This was someone who I had thought supported my career, who was enlightened enough to know that the way we experience the world can absolutely be shaped by gender and race and any other unchangeable characteristics. He was also someone who used to accidentally on purpose touch my butt when he was doing up my surgical gown so maybe I shouldn't have been so surprised that anyone pushing back against the status quo would be on his radar for all the wrong reasons.

Nearly a year after that fateful Christmas Day when Michelle died, for some reason, thoughts of her and all the

photos of her kids came rushing back into my consciousness. What had I given up by being a surgeon? What had
I sacrificed without knowing the gravity of that loss? I had
dedicated my life to helping other people, and more recently
to helping women, both as patients and for those hoping to
follow in my footsteps. I started to fear that I was not only
going to end up alone, as predicted, but that while things
may get better for those who came after me, I had made life
much harder for myself, professionally and personally.

In planning my career I had not once, not for a single
moment, factored in what my life outside surgery would look
like. It didn't matter; if I was a successful surgeon, that was
all the life I needed. In fact, even when my personal life went
to shit, I would bury my pain in work. Extra shifts, intense
study or running away to conferences far, far away cushioned
the blow of anything in the real world that upset me. To me,
surgery was my real life and the only one worth having, the
only one worth putting any effort into. I was so busy dedi-
cating everything I had to what I thought was my one true
love that I'd missed out on so much. And now I was terrified
that I had left it far too late. Not only that, but my relationship
with surgery had started to become one-sided, not unrequited
but more of a relationship that takes everything from you and
gives nothing in return.

Staring at my desk, the sadness hung over me, finally
asking the questions of myself that I should have asked years
ago. And like a filthy old habit, I pushed those feelings to
the side and started to tackle my perpetually overflowing

email, filled with the drudgery of administration, constant warnings that the hospital was, as usual, over capacity and patient letters. I opened one from a cardiologist; the subject line was the name of a lady whose aortic valve I had replaced a couple of months earlier in an emergency late one evening. She had done well and I thought, as I usually do, that some professional success would help to hide my personal fears.

'Currently, she is doing very well and has recovered nicely from surgery with return of normal heart function,' I read, the praise warming my heart, although that was to be short-lived. 'However, she is full of complaints including that a female did her surgery.' And with that dagger, the tears rushed free.

I had spent years of my life battling in a job that increasingly seemed like it would rather not have me there. The fear that I had given up too much for that job suddenly seemed overwhelming.

I was moping around the hospital. I went to see a new patient who had been referred to me.

'Dr Nikki!' she practically squealed. 'The nurse looking after me today said you were such a great surgeon *and* the only lady heart surgeon in the state. I have told everyone that I get the lady surgeon and I am so lucky and my grand-daughter can't wait to meet you.'

I could feel a lump at the back of my throat and I wanted to hug her.

I had needed to hear that more than she would ever know.

11

AUTUMN

Suspended in the cold

Even when you finish your training in medicine, your training is never actually finished. There is always something new to learn. A new procedure, a solution to a new problem, a new piece of technology. In the first few years of your practice, the learning curve seems incredibly steep. Rather than doing your procedures with someone else, suddenly you realise that you're the one in the room who is in charge.

But that doesn't mean you're alone, especially when, like me, you're at the start of your career as a consultant surgeon. When you're faced with one of these new situations, something you've never done before, you often work with senior colleagues to do procedures with their help.

I was going to be doing a huge operation, one that would take me at least six hours, using a device that I had never used before. It was going to involve the biggest blood vessel in the body, the aorta. I was going to have to replace the aorta from the heart, all the way down to the left side of the chest, where it curves like a walking cane to take blood all around the body. I'd have to disconnect some of the most important blood vessels in the body, including the coronary arteries and the arteries that supply blood to the head and neck.

If things went wrong I could ruin the heart, I could cause a stroke, I could make the patient a paraplegic or they could bleed to death. Not only that, it was a high-stakes surgery for the entire team, because to do all of this we would need to cool the patient down to just 20 degrees Celsius, a whole 17 degrees below normal body temperature. If you touched the patient during this time, you would be taken aback by how icy-cold their skin was.

I had done operations similar to this, but not exactly like this. And not while using a new device that would replace the most inaccessible end of the work that I was doing. I was a heady mix of excitement, because this was one of my favourite surgeries to do, and nerves, because as a young surgeon I felt like there was so much riding on it. This wasn't just a feeling: it was fact.

Although nobody said it, I knew that my reputation was on the line. In fact, every time I operated, I knew that was the case. When you have a good outcome, business continues as usual. When you have a bad outcome, whether it be because you made an error or because it wasn't your day, the vultures circle. And for female surgeons, the retribution is far greater. Research from Harvard University in 2017 has shown that if a woman surgeon has a death on her operating table other doctors refer to her less, a punishment that lasts for more than a year. There is no such effect for the men. And there is still less such effect if you're the experienced senior surgeon; they've earned the right to have bad outcomes.

Facing your colleagues after you've had a problem, even one that turned out well for the patient in the end, feels awful. Even as a junior doctor, I used to hear the way that doctors, and especially surgeons, would talk about their colleagues' complications. I once heard a surgeon describe another female surgeon as someone who should be kept away from sharp objects, after word got out that she had a particularly tough day at the office. Not letting someone operate on your dog was another charming way of commenting on a complication. The callousness with which we dealt with someone's misfortune (the patient's) and another's difficulties (our colleagues) was brutal. Although we're supposed to approach all our mistakes and those of others with curiosity and an openness to learn from them, we tended to make them a bit more of a witch-hunt than a learning opportunity.

I decided to ask a senior surgeon to help me with my big case with the shiny new device. I asked him because I didn't want the patient to bleed to death or have a massive stroke. I asked him because I wanted to learn from his experience. But, if I'm honest, I also wanted him there to insulate me from any insinuations that I wasn't good enough, especially if something went wrong.

He was one of my main teachers as I came up through the ranks. And he was hard on me. Every stitch had to be perfect. As I'd pass the needle through the vessel, he'd watch me like a hawk. 'No, no, no, no, yes, take that,' he'd say until I got the stitch in the absolutely correct position. There was no room for error and I loved that kind of teaching, although it was exhausting. I used to want to be just like him, surgically and in life. I wanted his swagger just as much as I wanted his technical ability.

Whenever I do a huge surgery like this, especially one that I don't do especially often, I make notes. Each step written out, complete with little diagrams of how to orient my instruments or the best way to set up the bypass circuit. I can close my eyes and see every step of the operation in my mind. I watch videos of other surgeons doing the same thing and study every letter of the patient's notes, every frame of their scans. I am so prepared that, by the time I get to the operating table, it feels like I've done the surgery ten times over before I even cut the skin.

With such a big case, there were more preparations to make than usual. There were extra lines to monitor nearly every function of the patient's body. The bypass machine needed some extra preparation and there were almost double the trays of shiny, silver instruments. Everyone's job got a bit more involved with big cases like this.

When we were eventually ready, I took my place at the patient's right-hand side and, with my registrar and nurse, began covering the patient head to toe in the sterile blue drapes that were going to keep him covered for however long this was going to take. Just like every other step of the surgery, this had to be perfect. Start as you mean to go on and all that.

When I opened the patient's chest and exposed the heart, the problem was plain to see. His aorta was massive, nearly twice as big as it should have been. When the aorta dilates, a condition called an aneurysm, the wall, usually thick and resilient, becomes very thin. Under the pressure of the heart pushing blood out along it, that thin aorta can tear or even rupture, an event we prefer to avoid. So we replace it before that terrible event can happen.

To keep the pipes from the heart–lung bypass machine out of the exact spot I'd be operating on, I connected the patient by making a small cut in his right groin. I still remember being absolutely enraged as a junior doctor by the spaghetti of pipes that connect to the bypass machine. They curl up over the operating field and half of the choreography of an operation is learning which way to rest the pipes so that they weren't in the way of your surgery. In an operation as taxing as this one, getting all of that out of the way was even more important.

Once the patient was safely in the hands of the perfusionist, we began to cool him down. Normal body temperature— 37 degrees Celcius—is the optimal temperature for the numerous chemical reactions that happen within our cells, all there to simply keep us alive. When we cool the body those chemical reactions slow down, using much less energy, as the cells are suspended in a kind of hibernation. While the whole body is protected by this, most importantly the slow-down protects the brain because, in not too long, I would basically be disconnecting the blood supply to his brain. Suffice to say, the stakes really couldn't have been higher.

Every now and again, I catch myself feeling a tiny bit of awe at what I'm about to do. It's not nerves; it's more a kind of astonishment at how far I've come. It seemed like only yesterday that simply putting stitches into simple wounds on the skin was something I had to learn to do. Now, I was about to reconstruct a man's entire aorta. It made me smile under my mask; whether it sounds arrogant or not I don't know, but I was really proud of the surgeon I had become.

As the patient's body temperature drifted down towards 20 degrees, I started the actual operation, just like I had imagined again and again in my mind. Clamp the aorta, transect the aorta, cut out the bottom, size a new replacement. Each step just as I had planned. When you have a surgery like this, once you start you simply cannot stop. One step must follow the next without so much as a pause because hibernation of the organs can't last forever. Once we're on that heart–lung bypass machine, once the aorta is in pieces, you just have to keep going.

One of the things I love about aortic surgery is the kilometres and kilometres of sutures. With a bright blue suture, I have to sew back together the aorta that I'm reconstructing. Each suture is like a life-and-death decision. One suture slightly out of place creates a leak, and when you leak five litres of blood a minute out of a hole it can be a serious problem. Of course, everything is checked and problems can be repaired (most of the time) but I always saw it as a challenge to make sure I never had to go back and fix any problems by putting in extra sutures. I wanted this to be perfect first time.

The next part of the surgery was the hardest, disconnecting, one by one, the blood vessels to the head. This is when the brain truly hibernates while it loses a huge chunk of its blood supply. The brain is exquisitely sensitive to losing its blood supply, so not only does this have to be done quickly, it has to be done well. The more there is riding on something I'm doing, the more I need to do it perfectly. Sometimes, at points like this in these surgeries, I can feel not only my own breath being held, but everyone else's too.

But breath holding wasn't needed, as much as I hated tempting fate by thinking that. I was beyond pleased with how everything was going. It was so smooth, just as I had imagined it.

The time had come to get my boss in. I know surgeons who would bristle at the idea of feeling like they needed help with something but I loved operating with my colleagues, especially my seniors. I had the rest of my career to carry the can alone, so I always saw any opportunity to have a second pair of hands and eyes and all that experience as a good thing. Even when I got to do cases with other specialties, I always learnt something. In my mind, surgery is a team sport and there is no real MVP, no star player.

Mr Swagger strolled into theatre in a grand entrance. I don't think this man had ever entered a room quietly in his life (actually, I'm sure of it). One piece of advice he gave me when I was a registrar was to always make sure people knew you were in the room. Ask questions, make comments and suggestions, let everyone know that you are there because the worst thing, in his opinion, is to be forgettable.

As per usual, his greeting was to the nurses, several of whom were happily pregnant.

'Hello, yummy mummies!'

Although I was concentrating, I managed to find a second to roll my eyes.

'I'm just about ready for you,' I told him. Ready to use this fancy new device. Aside from the pressure of using this new technology, this would be the highest stakes part of the surgery for another reason. For about twenty minutes, this man was about to have no circulation whatsoever. For want of a better term, we were about to switch him off completely.

It's a process called deep hypothermic circulatory arrest. At my word, once the patient's temperature was at 20 degrees, I'd tell the perfusionist to turn off the heart–lung machine. The perfusionist would then drain a large amount of blood from the patient back into the pump and, for nearly twenty minutes, not a single cell in the body would get fresh, oxygenated blood.

The reason we had to do this was that I had to join up the aorta to the replacement aorta deep down in the chest, just about at the spine. I would be operating down a deep dark hole, so to have the field filled with blood from the aorta would make it simply impossible. With every minute that ticked over, the risk of problems—strokes, spinal cord injury, kidney failure—started to climb precipitously. And since this was the part of the operation that used the new device, this is where our teamwork came in.

This position had been one I had been in for most of my training. Me on the patient's right side, doing the operation. My boss, my mentor, my friend, opposite me, shepherding me through some complex skill. Things had changed a lot now, especially since Mr Swagger no longer had to adjudicate every suture like he did when I first started learning. Now we were supposed to be peers in some aspects but, more importantly, it was always intimated that I was going to be passed the torch from him. I had always thought of him as the type of mentor who knows that you will grow and improve over time. Actually, I thought of him as the type of great mentor who would hope that I would excel above him one day.

We got ready to go. Everyone in the theatre fell into a hushed silence because this was when everyone's concentration had to be at its highest. Mr Swagger and I checked and double-checked everything—our device, our sutures, our instruments. The aorta was prepared so that as soon as the pumped turned off, I could go like the wind. The anaesthetists had packed the patient's head in ice, to keep the brain even cooler, and given him a medication to slow the brain's activity even further so it wouldn't use what precious energy it did have, accidentally starving itself.

'Everybody ready to turn off?' I asked the whole theatre. As everyone in turn agreed, I said again, 'Okay, Stu, come off, please. And let me know every five minutes, thanks.'

As the perfusionist slowly drained the patient, I started this time-critical part of the operation, transecting the aorta at the back of the chest, trimming, measuring, making sure that everything was perfect. My boss across from me would occasionally chime in with encouragement or little suggestions.

I put my hand out for the new device I was going to use, which my scrub nurse handed up to me. In time crunches like this, the scrub nurse knowing exactly what you want is a literal godsend.

'Five minutes.'

We were right on time. In the last five minutes, I wasn't sure I had looked up at all. Every second I was working, doing something to get this critical part of the surgery done. The clock is always ticking in heart surgery, but never more than it was now. I lined up the graft to be able to reconnect the aorta and resume delivery of blood to the body and started sewing, every stitch needing to be perfect more than ever because if this bled later, I would struggle to be able to get in there to fix it.

'Ten minutes.'

Over halfway. Although I was still going well, we were over halfway. My boss reassured me; maybe he picked up on the fact that we had a paltry ten minutes left to sew this aorta back together with the graft. Not that there was time to consciously register that I was feeling pressure, but I knew that it was there. I knew, even it was deep down, that if I screwed this up, the consequences were dire.

'Fifteen minutes.'

The last suture was going in just as the fifteen-minute call came. Now all I had to do was connect the new aorta to the machine so that we could restore blood flow before that dreaded twenty-minute mark. Trying not to get white line fever—celebrating before the job was actually done—I re-arranged the pipes of the heart–lung bypass machine, plugging them in and preparing to turn the pump back on and, in a way, turn the patient back on too.

'You can slowly start coming on, Stu,' I said to the perfusionist, to start delivering blood back to the patient. We want to turn everything on slowly, so as not to make a mess with an enormous gush of blood but also to let the lifegiving fluid slowly seep into every space that we had just drained it from.

I watched my newly formed suture line, making sure it didn't spring a leak as the blood started flowing past it. It's at times like this that you're better off not marvelling at how a thin layer of thread is somehow able to hold together the full force of the circulatory system. If you start thinking about it, it's scary.

'Come back up to full flow and start rewarming.'

I had done it, the most difficult part of the surgery. And it looked perfect. I asked the perfusionist how long we had been switched off for.

Eighteen minutes.

How unbelievable: this man was in a state of limbo for eighteen whole minutes. I was thrilled at the incredible nature of the human body and the technology we had to do this, as well as the fact that I had had two whole minutes to spare.

'Not bad, doc,' Mr Swagger said to me. 'Almost as good as me; I did it in seventeen last week.'

I rolled my eyes in jest and teased him for turning everything into a competition. 'Everything *is* a competition, doc,' he said back. 'We're not here training for the easy ones.' And with that bit of sage advice he unscrubbed, shouting 'Call me if you need a hand,' as the door to theatre swung shut.

The operation took another couple of hours to complete. Rewarming someone from 20 degrees Celcius back up to the normal 37 degrees Celcius takes time and it takes precision. Doing it too quickly can cause almost as much damage as anything else that we do. Not to mention that getting every cell back to this important level is simply a process that is bound by the laws of physics. Despite the hard parts being over, there was much work to do: putting every part back together, checking every suture line, every hole we made. Making sure the heart worked after its prolonged slumber, making sure there was no bleeding, making sure everything was perfect.

As the end of the surgery approached, I started to notice my back crying out. Although I am tall, the operating table I needed specifically for this kind of surgery was too high for me. Even lowered down as far as it would go, I still had to stand on a step that was unforgiving on my legs and back.

These kinds of things were common for female surgeons; theatres and instruments were designed for men who were most often taller and had larger hands. My 1.7-metre (5 foot 7) height and petite hands just had to deal with the cards that we were dealt.

Although I was uncomfortable and hungry, the fact that I had a moment to think about my own body for a second was a good sign. It meant that the end of the operation was nigh and I no longer needed to be as hyper-focused on avoiding problems. It was like the rest of the world, shut out for several hours, could finally come back into view. I looked up at the clock, realising that the last six hours had seemed like they had flown by. Long surgeries were like that—you could quite literally get lost in them.

With the skin closed and the patient getting ready to go back to ICU, I sat down in the tiny room next to theatre where I could still watch everything going on but my tired back and legs could have a reprieve. My boss rounded the corner and surveyed the situation.

'I was just coming down to see if you'd finished yet,' he said, asking me how everything ended up. I told him it had looked great.

Mr Swagger took the seat next to me and wheeled in close in a way that made me uncomfortable. In the fifteen years I had known this man, he had had absolutely no idea about personal space. My knee was dangerously close to his groin.

'I know it's been a hard year for you,' he started. He was right. I had been increasingly unable to hide the immense pressure that this workplace was doling out to me. But I didn't know if his remark was empathy and solidarity or a slight. It felt more like the latter than the former. Either way, I could feel emotions starting to rise and trying to break free as tears.

'You're a very talented surgeon, Nik; you've just proved that. Not everyone can do what you've just done.'

The fact that he was making me feel all kinds of uncomfortable by his very unwelcome and inappropriately intimate invasion of my space vanished for just a second and all I wanted to do was sob. I was so happy with what we had all just done and immensely proud. Not only that, but I had loved that surgery. It made me feel alive.

The problem was that outside the little world that actually doing a heart surgery created in my head, being a surgeon was feeling more and more about keeping my head above water. It was starting to feel like I was fighting for my own survival as much as for my patient's.

* * *

If I could sum up my career in one sentence, it would be that I was always having to prove myself. And I don't think that's just me. From very early on, there is a never-ending series of tests that you have to pass to prove your worthiness as a doctor. Some of the tests are legitimate, like exams, designed to test your skill and knowledge. Some, though, are designed to simply test you personally.

It probably comes as no surprise that as a group, surgeons can be incredibly competitive. After all, getting into medical school is hard. Getting into a specialty training program even harder. Surviving that program is a feat, with excellent doctors quitting every year. This is the kind of competitiveness that might broadly be seen as a good thing. After all, I've been a patient on an operating table and I wanted the best of the best, right? Not someone who just scraped through.

I still remember, as a registrar in plastic surgery, one of my consultants bragging about how he would regularly 'break' the junior doctors. Not through a selection of carefully curated tests to see who had the best skills or the best bedside manner. He wasn't looking for the best or brightest by any metric that would be considered acceptable. Instead, he terrorised us with sleepless nights and constant berating. As each person would slowly drop out, buckling under the pressure of being treated like shit, not the job, he'd gleefully claim that he'd 'broken another one'.

We tell ourselves we're weeding out the weak for the benefit of society at large. And while that may be true in some cases, the gatekeeping and competitiveness that goes on actually seems more about protecting reputations as the top dogs and the bottom lines of lucrative private practices. Consultant surgeons act like bouncers at an exclusive nightclub, choosing who gets to make it and be successful and who gets to fade into insignificance, sometimes actively pushing them to do so.

Not long after this patient's aorta was pieced back together, I was trying to build my private practice. Many surgeons in

Australia have a dual private and public practice, working a few days a week in our publicly funded teaching hospitals and another few days a week in private practice. Building a private practice is hard, hard work where the competitiveness seems to ramp up, because now there is money involved.

I still remember the heady excitement of my very first private referral. One of my favourite cardiologists tracked me down in the hospital one day. He was my favourite, principally because he was an excellent clinician who time and time again went above and beyond for his patients. He was also averse to nonsense, a trait we shared that sometimes landed me in hot water.

'I've noticed how hard you've been working lately, so I thought I'd refer you this case as a bit of a reward.' Now, I know he meant well but it felt so odd, like I had finally cleared some invisible hurdle and been deemed worthy, based on working my tail off, to be ready to work more. Nonetheless, I was excited to stick a toe in the door of private practice. Not for its riches; all I had heard in that exchange was that, finally, someone thought I was good enough in some aspect.

Over the preceding year or so, I had started to wonder if I was. Not on paper, because on paper I was working hard, performing lots of surgeries. I was sticking my hand up to help out whenever I was needed and taking on extra work of all kinds. My outcomes were good; my patients did well. But I still desperately felt like I didn't belong. I still felt like I was the odd man out.

I started to have a trickle of private cases referred to me, all with the same sentiment as my favourite cardiologist: I had done enough to deserve this. I was being welcomed into some kind of club where the powers that be had decided I was worthy enough to be tapped on the shoulder.

My mentor had been letting me use his private rooms a couple of times and his secretary was helping me out with the administrative side of running a business, which is essentially what this was. Starting out was not only daunting, it was expensive. Generally, when you're a younger surgeon, this is a rite of passage that the older surgeons help you through. They take you under their wing, invite you to join their practice and help you get started. It's the collegiate way to do it.

I decided that I wanted to be able to take on more private patients and build a business of my own. Which meant that I would have to get up the courage to ask to join Mr Swagger's practice on a more permanent basis. I feel like this would be akin to asking for a raise in the corporate world. I really needed his help, as much as I had needed his help to tackle a complex operation that I hadn't a tonne of experience in. This was what a mentor was supposed to do, right?

I had my bravery dialled up as far as it would go as I marched into our department office at the public hospital, ready to ask for help. Our office was bare; nobody was around. Had I missed something? Was an emergency happening? I noticed the door to our conference room was closed and opened it just a crack to see if they were there. And there they all were, the other consultants, having a meeting. A meeting that nobody had told me about.

They all looked up at me like I was an intruder. Consultant meetings were not only sacred, they were a rite of passage. An invitation to an inner sanctum where the grown-ups would talk about the direction of the unit and high-level problems, and gain insights into the things that were considered too sensitive for little ears. As it dawned on them that they had forgotten about me, there was a chorus of grown men half-heartedly apologising for excluding me. Again. Being left out of the inner sanctum was becoming a frequent occurrence.

I sheepishly asked to come in and take my seat at the table, where I spent the remaining five minutes of the meeting feeling embarrassed rather than paying attention to the conversation at hand. My bravery to ask for help was all of a sudden vanishing.

As the meeting ended, I asked my mentor if he had a minute to talk about something else. Voice shaking, I told him that I had started getting a few private referrals.

He smirked. 'Well, I'd better put a stop to that!' He was joking. At least I think he was joking. Given that I had just been excluded from a meeting, I briefly wondered whether he might not have been. I shook my head and silently berated myself for thinking such a thing.

I explained to him how I needed his help to get started in my own private practice, just like everyone else had before. And as my mentor, and hopefully my friend, he was naturally the person I wanted to ask.

He began to explain how he had always thought I would be the person to take over his practice, his position, one day. 'After all,' he explained, 'we do the same work, like that aortic bloke,' mentioning the case he had helped me with a few weeks ago.

I could feel my heart racing with excitement, thinking I was about to get the medical equivalent of a raise or a promotion. How I was going to get to work side by side with the man who had taught me how to be a surgeon, not just in the operating theatre but who had inspired me to walk with the same swagger he did.

He asked if I had any other options. I told him I supposed I could go and get my own rooms. He doodled on the page in front of him and looked thoughtful for a moment, and I expected him to say that he wouldn't hear of such a thing. That, as his protegée, I should take my rightful place in the line of succession.

'I think that would be a really good idea.'

I had just been rejected and it felt like I had been stabbed right in the heart. I had no idea what had just happened. A few weeks ago, I was a talented surgeon. A few moments ago, I was next in line to the throne. I thought that I had jumped through every hoop imaginable but it turns out that I hadn't.

Almost every day, it seemed, these guys were thinking of new ways to tell me that I didn't belong. For a job that I loved because of the way it was a team sport and that we were all in it together, I had never felt more alone.

12

EASTER

God is not a cardiothoracic surgeon

'Whatever you reckon, doc.'

I bristle whenever patients say that to me. It makes me feel uncomfortable that they appear, at least, to be handing over all of their autonomy to me and what I think is best for them. I'm trying to condense all of my knowledge, and often the collective knowledge, wisdom and experience of many of my peers and decades of research, into a 40-minute consultation that is supposed to meld that knowledge together with the person's hopes and values. Not only that, we're both trying to predict the future with an outcome that is everything they want and need. It feels very god-like, and not in a good way, to have that influence over someone.

I'd spent so much time with this man over the previous couple of days. He had one of the most feared and unusual complications of a heart attack, called an infarct ventricular septal defect (VSD for short). When you have a heart attack, unless we can restore blood flow to the heart muscle quickly, that part of the heart dies. And when heart muscle dies, it can't regenerate; the heart is one of the few organs in the body that can never grow back. You can cut out half of your liver and it will grow back. Skin will heal. Even your blood cells turn over and renew every few weeks. Your heart, though, that's it; you only have one.

When the heart muscle dies, the dead muscle cells almost dissolve in a process called liquefaction. The once-strong muscle becomes mushy, and under the pressure of the blood in the heart the mushy heart muscle gives way to a hole. And in the case of a VSD, that hole occurs in the septum (the wall) dividing the left and right ventricles. Blood then goes from the high-pressure left ventricle to the low-pressure right side, making the patient deathly unwell most of the time. It's a condition that has a high mortality rate without surgery but, even with surgery, the outcome can be just as grim.

When I first met this patient, he was unwell but not knocking on death's door. He didn't want surgery; in fact, he was adamant that he just wanted to go home and die. I spent so much time just chatting to him, about his life, what he did with his free time, his grandkids and how much he loved fishing. And each time I said to him, 'You know you're very sick, right? You might die.'

Every time, he responded, 'Yeah, love, but at least I won't die here.' Dying in hospital, connected to machines, away from your space and the people you love, is most folks' worst nightmare.

After a day and a half of hanging on, things took a turn for the worse. He started to have trouble breathing and his blood pressure was getting lower. His kidneys, lacking blood supply, started to show signs of failing. What had likely happened was, despite all of our treatment, the mushy heart muscle was giving rise to a bigger and bigger hole and the heart was not happy about it, struggling to pump. It was now or never. This was to have been a high-risk surgery to start with; now it was extremely high risk. I rang two of my senior colleagues, one in Sydney, for advice to see if we had missed the boat and I should honour his original wishes or whether we should just go to theatre now and try to fix the hole. They both said resoundingly, do it now or don't do it at all.

I went into his room and laid everything on the table, basically saying that he wasn't going to make it home. We could operate now and hope for the best but, realistically, he had at best a fifty-fifty chance of making it. That wasn't a wild guess either; we have risk calculators, where you plug in patient variables like how old they are and what surgery they're having, that take hundreds of thousands of patients' data from many decades to spew out a number that says how likely it is that person will live or die. The calculator told me his risk of dying was 31.48 per cent, but since it often underestimates these situations I painted a much more desperate picture.

'What do I do, doc?' he asked me, seemingly putting the decision firmly in my hands.

I hesitated for a moment, trying to disentangle my feelings as a human who wants to make things better no matter what from those as a doctor, whose job it is to carefully weigh things in an unemotional manner to do the best for that patient. I said, 'We need to give it a shot, I think,' but deep down I knew that it might not have been the right answer.

Given how sick the man was, I asked one of my senior colleagues to help with the surgery. Serious cases like this are not the time for showing off and feeding our egos. They need everything we can throw at them, and that includes as many experienced hands as we can find.

With the heart quiet on bypass, we turned it upside down to see the back where the heart attack had occurred. I cut into the area the heart attack had affected (so as not to put a cut through much needed healthy heart muscle); the heart was so soft and abnormal, I felt sick at how damaged it was. I had been expecting a small hole on the inside, in the septum, but it was so much worse than that. The hole was massive and that feeling of sickness intensified; I had known the odds were not in our favour to begin with and now they were lengthening even further.

We patched the septum with a piece of Dacron (a synthetic fabric we use to reconstruct many things), but each time I pushed my needle through the supposedly healthy muscle to anchor the patch, it too was so damaged that it couldn't hold the stitch and the suture just pulled through. I did that patch twice before I thought we might have had a win and closed the hole. Eventually, we managed to patch the hole closed.

For a second, I wondered if we might have succeeded and I felt a rush of excitement—what if he survived? I even went as far as to let myself think that we had done the impossible. Before then, though, I had to close the hole in the outside of the heart that we had used to access the septum, but it too had the same problem: it was so damaged.

Hours dragged by as we tried every trick we could think of to close the heart. But nothing was working; blood kept coming from the hole in the back of the heart. His body was falling apart; the heart, the kidneys, his blood pressure was difficult to maintain. Everything kept going from bad to worse to eventually completely irretrievable. After many hours and the input of not just the two surgeons at the table but the entire theatre team, ICU and another colleague on the phone, he died alone on the cold, hard operating table. When the machines get turned off, to quiet the alarms and pings telling us that things aren't going well, it's a painful silence, like a symbol of the finality of what has just occurred.

I was devastated. I'm always devastated when a patient dies but this one stung more than others. Because he hadn't wanted this operation, not really. He had only agreed to it when he was absolutely petrified, after his body began shutting down and an endless stream of doctors (myself included) and nurses reassured him that this was the only way we could save his life, even though we all said it was a long shot. But it was ultimately me, as the surgeon, telling him that he would certainly die without an operation, but he might survive with one. And in that intense fear, he'd deferred to me to act like a god and save his life against all the odds. In the last few days of his life, he'd told me that he hadn't wanted to die at hospital. And in the end, that's exactly what had happened.

'I never should have done this operation,' I told one of my senior colleagues on the phone. 'I'll never know if he really wanted to give this operation a shot or if he just wanted to die peacefully.' I could feel the tears start to roll down my cheeks as I concentrated on not overtly bawling my eyes out, lest I be seen as unprofessional and over-emotional.

'You did what you thought was right and you did what the patient said,' he said, which put me at ease a little bit. But then, he said, 'You know, if it had been someone like me operating, maybe it would have been a different outcome.' That made me screw up my face in confusion and irritation in equal measures. I was hurting and that was just another kick in the teeth.

My colleague who had come to help with the surgery found me as I was reeling from both the outcome of the surgery and the less-than-supportive phone call. I told him the same thing: I think I may have made the wrong call to operate here.

Thankfully, his emotional intelligence is higher than that of many others. 'Look, maybe, but you're never going to know that. The guy wanted surgery; he wanted a chance and this was his only chance. Had we known just how horrific it was going to be, yeah, we might have made a different call but he had a one hundred per cent chance of dying without surgery and he wanted you to try to take whatever possibility of success and give it a go. And you did a good job; you did a good operation.'

I felt better but not brilliant. 'But if it hadn't been me operating, if it had been someone else . . .' I told him what our colleague had said, all the way from across the country where he was doing his calm elective list with no hearts that were falling apart.

'What, does he think he's God or something? Nobody could have saved that. Probably not even God. That guy—' He rolled his eyes. 'Next, he'll tell you he's walking on water.'

The strangeness of this situation was that I felt like I had been asked to play God by making that tough call. Had we saved that man's life, against the odds, maybe I would have felt at least lucky or even like we did a good job. Instead, I was left feeling like I had been asked to be some sort of miracle worker and I was never, ever going to be able to measure up to that. Surgery isn't a miracle and surgeons aren't gods or miracle workers; we're just here to give our bodies a head start at fighting off the enemy. While some of us might feel comfortable or even relish accepting the mantle of an omnipotent being, that was never going to be the way I felt. I am always acutely aware of the fallibility of humans and of my own fallibility in particular. Being asked to play God or being among those who want to makes me feel uncomfortable to my very core.

I couldn't help but wonder: is that a failing as a surgeon? Not actually being a miracle worker or failing to act like one could be equally seen as weaknesses. Yet I could do something about only one of those.

***

There's a joke about nearly every specialty in medicine, designed to poke fun at the stereotypes of that particular group of doctors. We recite them about orthopaedic surgeons, oncologists, you name it. And they're funny not because they're particularly witty but because they're worryingly accurate portrayals of the shortcomings of that group.

The standard joke about heart surgeons is:

Q: What's the difference between God and a cardiothoracic surgeon?
A: God doesn't think he's a cardiothoracic surgeon.

I can assure you that this joke is not meant as a compliment to the extraordinary skill of surgeons; rather, it's a pointed barb about the infamous surgeon's ego. Everyone has heard of a surgeon's ego. Some of us have even been unlucky enough to experience the dark side of this confidence so great that it elevates its owner above even omnipotent beings.

As part of my surgical training, I had to do quite a lot of time in ICU. It was meant to teach us the finer points of treating critically unwell patients. Now I wonder if it was also there to humble us, to help us understand the point of view of our colleagues and develop a profound respect for what they do. My time in ICU was all of those things for me. A time to learn more to make myself a better doctor and a time when I saw myself and my colleagues in a different light.

During my ICU rotation, we had to place a central line in a patient who was critically unwell. I was very attached to this patient, partly because he was so young, barely out of his teens, but also because he had been admitted with severe heart failure, which of course sat well with my fascination with all things heart. To place a central line, the tube breaches the skin, travels through the vein and sits just at the entrance of the heart. This line can get infected and cause life-threatening sepsis to patients; because of that, we take extraordinary steps to ensure that the line is inserted in a sterile fashion. The patient is painted with antiseptic, covered in drapes and the line itself is impregnated with an antibiotic to stop bugs growing on it. When we put these lines in we all wear surgical gloves, a surgical gown, a mask and a hat to cover the hair.

The patient's mother was there, in her mask and hat, holding her son's hand, trying to help him through the fact that in just a few days, his whole world had come crashing down in ways many of us could never imagine. I was going to be putting the line in. As I'd only done this line half a dozen times, the ICU consultant was there helping me. I was about to start when a consultant surgeon flung the door open and walked in: no mask, no hat. He started talking to the patient, who was underneath the drapes. He barely acknowledged the patient's mother (who happened to be a nurse) in the corner or his colleague, the ICU consultant, and he definitely ignored the standards for infection control that we were all observing. The patient's mother piped up from the corner, 'Excuse me, who are you and why aren't you wearing a hat like everyone else? They're putting in a central line.'

He turned to her and said, 'I'm the surgeon and the rules don't apply to me. Plus, I never get infections. Ever.' And then he snickered.

That is where these jokes come from. From the extraordinary ego that allows flaunting of the rules with wild abandon, safe in the knowledge that nobody will ever hold you accountable because you're just so good.

The problem with the surgeon's ego is that it can be outright destructive. Far too many patients have been on the receiving end of the all-knowing surgeon, who acts like we still practise medicine in the days when patients would defer to them with a simple, 'Whatever you think is best, doctor.'

Times have changed. Especially in recent years, we have seen a shift away from the power of the doctor to the unwavering primacy of the patient. And rightly so. What I need is, and should be, dwarfed by the patient's needs and wants. The surgeon's ego has absolutely no place when it comes to patients. Despite this push to make surgeons more kind, more inclusive and less egotistical, patients are still sadly subjected to the overblown self-esteem of a surgeon from time to time. We've all experienced it or read about it—doctors who inflict their views on patients, speak to them disparagingly or dismiss their experience.

Patients are not the only ones on the receiving end of our misconceptions about our place in the hierarchy. If people ever think that surgeons inflict their hubris on patients alone, you should see how we treat each other. We fight over who is best, turning green with envy when another surgeon's abilities are lauded. To junior staff and colleagues, surgeons behave like they are the hand of Benediction, choosing who will be successful and who won't. Surgeons have, for decades, sued each other for restricting their practice when one makes defamatory comments about another. We select our trainees, our future colleagues, but ensure that we maintain just enough control over them in their careers, and even in their lives, so that they can only progress with our divine blessing. As one of my former bosses used to say, 'When you get a good reference from me, people know it really means something,' as if he alone chose who would rise through the ranks to one day take a place upon high. Sometimes I wonder if surgeons enjoy exerting power over each other even far more than over patients.

I find it really hard to believe that there are that many natural narcissists in the world. Surgery may well attract people who are confident, perhaps even arrogant, but these traits are rewarded and nurtured to grow some into monstrosities. We place a group of achievement-oriented people who are probably perfectionists by nature in a highly competitive environment where perfectionism and overconfidence are rewarded and dissociation from emotion is, at least some-times, necessary. Doctors and surgeons are bred in a system that unheedingly takes traits that make us good at our jobs and amplifies them until they are pathological.

We have been inadvertently taught that we are the only profession that can truly do good in the world, the only ones who can truly save lives or make a difference in people's lives. We get to come into the most dire situations and save the day, and we get to bask in the glory of doing so. I don't think that this is intentional; doctors and surgeons are held in such high esteem, and often with good reason. But it feeds into this idea that we are truly gifted or truly special, and we then risk spending our entire careers—entire lives—trying to be even more so. We spend every waking moment chasing an ideal that we can never, ever reach. Surgeons have long been put on a pedestal; at times, it's hard to imagine that this kind of worship hasn't led to an entire profession developing a psychopathy. The biggest sign of our morality is what we do with power, and the way we wield that power on each other is truly telling.

This idea of ego, of god complexes, is not just in my imag-ination. Many research studies have confirmed that surgeons tend to score particularly high on markers of narcissism. More worrying research has shown that egotistical behaviours pose a genuine threat to the wellbeing of patients and staff alike, which is why, starting at medical school, such behaviours are now being excised, training the new generation of doctors to check their god complex at the door. But the system still stokes the development of the pathological ego by allowing surgeons with delusions of grandeur to flaunt the rules, like the one in my ICU rotation, or rewarding bad behaviour by excusing their missteps on account of their prowess in the operating room. All is forgiven if you can cure with your own hands. Recent years have seen an explosion of courses and compulsory training designed to bring surgeons back to earth, not a moment too soon. Sometimes, as I watch the grandiosity around me, I wonder if it is all in vain though.

At the same time, I can't let go of the sense that surgery is not a game for the meek of heart. I think there is a degree of necessary egotism running through the veins of every surgeon. An unshakable belief that you can and will succeed. A confidence that quietens the social more that it's not okay to inflict pain on another person, even if it is for their good. I know that when I stand on the right-hand side of some-one's chest, I'm not there to be mediocre. I'm there to do a brilliant job and I know that I can. I *have* to think that.

Sawing open someone's sternum, holding someone's heart in your hands, making split-second life-or-death calls? Not only does that take knowledge, skill and decisiveness, it takes a huge dose of confidence in yourself: an unwavering belief that you can violate someone's very being, go inside and triumph. And that is the story we're told from very early on: that to be a surgeon you need to be god-like, because what we do to people, where we have trodden, only deities have gone before us. Anything that can help you emulate that level of divinity—the way you walk, the way you talk, the person that you are—is erroneously considered to be synonymous with your ability as a surgeon.

I remember sitting in the tearoom, about to start surgery on a patient. She needed a Bentall's procedure—a big operation, even by heart-surgery standards, where we replace the aortic valve, the first part of the aorta, and reimplant the coronary arteries, akin to taking the heart apart and putting it back together. It's not an operation for the faint of heart and I don't know what it says about me that it's my favourite surgery to perform. I sat there looking at her scans one last time, going through what needed to be done and how I would do it in my head.

For some reason, my surgeon's ego was absent that day. This wave of uncertainty washed over me as I started to wonder what right I had to be performing this major surgery on this woman. For a second, I even entertained the idea of cancelling, sending her off to another surgeon. Someone who wasn't sitting there before surgery doubting their ability. I still, to this day, don't know what it was that caused me to think like that. I don't even know if other surgeons' confidence has ever faltered like that, because nobody ever talks about it. I found my ego, my confidence, and trusted my ability to do the procedure and everything was fine. I went home and bragged about how well things had gone, lest anyone suspect for a moment I had doubted I was the superhuman I was supposed to be.

There really isn't a place for a lack of confidence or a lack of belief in surgery. At least, that's what I had always thought. Now I don't know how true that is. Decades of watching surgeons swagger down hallways like they owned the place, of bravado, had taught me that this is the only way to be a surgeon—with the absolute belief that you were God, or as close as is humanly possible.

I wonder what seeing things like that did to me, an impressionable young doctor who wanted to be a surgeon, who wanted to emulate great doctors. That surgeon from my ICU term, in particular: I was absolutely in awe of him and his abilities. I used to hope that I could be half as good as he was. Did that give me and many others who witnessed similar things the idea that overconfidence is a quality found in accomplished surgeons? That breaking the rules and not being accountable is an important facet of being a successful and respected surgeon.

After my patient with the VSD died, I thought a lot about ego and god complexes in surgeons. I thought a lot about the supposed divinity of surgeons. Would my patient have survived if someone closer to a divine being than me had operated? Even though, logically, I know that this is likely not the case—that his illness was too great for anyone to repair—I couldn't escape the thought that my interstate colleague had implanted in my head. That maybe, when the situation is that dire, you really do need to be touched by the hand of God.

More importantly, that patient made me ruminate on a much more important question, a bigger worry. Would my ego lead me to make the wrong call about someone? Had it led me to make the wrong call in his case, by choosing to try my hand at being God and fighting against the odds for a miracle in a situation that was seemingly unwinnable? I can say with all honesty that I didn't choose to operate on that man on that day to prove anything. I didn't decide that I had the biggest balls and wasn't afraid to take on a risky case. I did it because I wanted to save him; I wanted to give him a chance at life.

I wrestled with this for a long time, wondering if I had done the wrong thing and whether his fear of dying had triggered in me an intense need to perform a miracle. After much soul searching and deep discussion with colleagues who lacked a pathological god complex, I concluded I had done the right thing. But I cannot stop thinking about how the god complex of a surgeon is not a thing to be revered, but rather something to be tamed. Confidence should be used to meet the needs of a vulnerable and fearful patient, not to prove that you are the best or to exert influence over your colleagues in a way that is nothing short of damaging. If saving lives is performing miracles, I think that is a wonderful and noble part of our profession. But our hubris can be our undoing, damaging our patients, each other and our own minds. It dawned on me that I might wrestle to balance confidence and hubris for my whole career. And in the spirit of all things godly, I can only pray that I get the balance right.

13

WINTER

Heart and soul

God, I was tired. My colleagues had all booked holidays at the same time, leaving me and one other colleague to do the work of five surgeons. The unit was only supposed to allow one or two of us away at a time and you were supposed to actually communicate with each other and negotiate who would go when. But that would involve compromise, not our strong suit. Either way, the lack of other surgeons and increased workload had left me annoyed and tired, never a good combination.

The fact that we were lacking in manpower meant I had been operating pretty much nonstop for several days. One emergency had kept me at work until late two nights earlier and, as that patient struggled through the night, the regular phone calls from my registrar and the intensive care doctors to keep me updated of my patient's progress meant I hadn't had much sleep and I hadn't recovered from the deficit. It also meant I hadn't done all the things that keep me healthy and sane, like going for a run or eating a meal that contains actual vegetables, rather than one that came from a vending machine and would survive nuclear fallout.

I honestly felt like my eyes were about to fall out of my head, I was so unbelievably tired. When I was a registrar, it was a rite of passage that we all had to go through, working and operating on virtually zero sleep. At worst, some jobs saw me working in excess of eighty hours a week. Even when you were so tired you couldn't even remember your own name you still came to work, either because you were instructed to or because you dared not catch up on sleep. I was very familiar with why sleep deprivation is used as a method of torture.

I will never forget being awake for nearly 48 hours for one operation as a registrar. It is a pain that is seared into my brain and makes my heart beat fast just to think about it. We started operating at 8 a.m. on Thursday, finished at 4 a.m. on Friday and then, as the patient had a complication, raced her back to theatre just one hour later. I got home that Friday evening at 6 p.m., having asked my mother to pick me up from the hospital because I was too tired to drive safely. Not too tired to operate, though; that was fine.

I always found the ritual sleep deprivation torture to be inhumane, but I was determined never to be broken by it. As a result, I can nap pretty much anywhere. I've slept in the back of police cars while sirens blared on transplant runs, on the floor of operating theatres, in my car, in the library, under a desk or—my personal favourite in summer—on the balcony outside ICU, which was more romantic than it sounds because at least it was under the stars.

The thing is, I always agreed that sleep deprivation was a necessity. As one of my former bosses told me, you need to know how to operate when you're tired. He was right. It shouldn't be par for the course but someone is going to come crashing through the door one night when you're already exhausted or it's the wee small hours and their life depends on you being compos mentis enough to do your job.

But I could never get on board with the ritualised and forced sleeplessness as a marker of worthiness or being tough enough. As a consultant, I made a point of trying to do better for myself and my registrars. But there was always a pang of guilt when I retreated to rest and recuperate, like I wasn't tough enough. Or I wasn't hardening my registrars enough.

As junior doctors, we always seemed especially vulnerable. You were in this survival game where you were constantly competing to be accepted—into training programs if you were not yet a training registrar, to different jobs around the country, passing exams and even just to be liked or treated well by those around you.

In 2010, a survey from Australian mental health charity Beyond Blue revealed atrocious statistics about the mental health of doctors, with one in ten reporting thoughts of suicide in the previous year and a rate of anxiety and depression far in excess of the general population or of other professions.

I've lost far too many colleagues and friends to suicide and watched many more suffer in silence, afraid to face the stigma of being a doctor who needs help. You see, we're not supposed to need help. We're okay to be giving help to others but if you're the one with panic attacks or the one who can't get out of bed, that's not okay. The stigma follows you around, from your own judgement and sometimes from your colleagues who might say that you're just not cut out for being a surgeon if you can't hold it together.

Added to all of this, doctors were beholden to something called mandatory reporting. This basically meant that if I went to my doctor complaining of an illness that could impact my work, they would have to report me to the medical board or else we could both risk losing our registration. Among the reportable conditions was mental illness, and as a result doctors were left to believe that they would be deregistered if they sought help, losing everything that they'd worked most of their lives for. Updates to these requirements in recent times now allow doctors to seek care without losing their careers, but that fear still persists. Reporting isn't the only way to destroy a career—stigma can have a similar effect.

These genuine threats to the lives of doctors were swept under the carpet. Anyone who was suffering with burnout or worse was explained away as just not being cut out for the job. They weren't tough enough. It had nothing to do with the cesspool we were expected to work in, the constant sacrifice. It was that we were not resilient enough. Or that we didn't know how to relax.

None of that was a new problem but it took a string of doctor suicides to get media attention to force hospitals and professional colleges to at least appear to be doing something. And so came an endless array of 'wellbeing measures' designed to perk us up.

The problem of doctor burnout or mental illness had nothing to do with a lack of wellness programs, but rather the fact that we marinate in other people's misery or that we're totally sleep deprived and increasingly lack job security. It also went without saying that the sexism, the bullying or the endless list of problems largely perpetrated by our employers and seniors didn't help either. Hospitals always seem to think the cure-all will be one of two things: yoga or resilience training.

It's much easier to schedule some yoga classes, usually in the middle of the day when we're at our busiest, rather than address the systemic issues at hand. I'm not without sympathy; fixing every issue in the healthcare system would be hard. Systemic issues aside, dealing with life or death, quite literally, wears everyone down to some degree. In my mind, though, the fact that this job is hard enough without all the other factors is even more reason to take proper care of each and every one of us.

Midway through my hell week, I finally got some sleep; the week that felt like it was never going to end was finally ending. And since I had gotten some sleep, I sprang out of bed at 5 a.m. with an unshakable desire for a run. A run would clear my head, strengthen my body and make me grateful for 40 minutes all to myself. Nothing but the sound of my feet on the pavement and my breath fogging up the air in front of me. It was cold but I loved the icy feeling on my face—it was invigorating, and if ever I needed to be re-energised it was now.

I was just 500 metres down the road when the phone rang, the hospital number flashing up. 'Hi, doctor, switchboard here. We have the emergency department on the line.' Shit. When ED calls the consultant directly, it's not usually a good sign.

I stopped running and panted, 'No worries, pop them through.'

The calmest voice in the universe came through the speaker. 'Hi, I'm the ED registrar on, are you the cardiothoracic surgeon?'

I affirmed that I was, nervously waiting to hear what he was calling me about.

'There's a 30-year-old man that the radiographer called a code blue on while he was in the scanner.' A radiographer is the medical scientist who runs the machines like the CT scanner or the MRI scanner and they get annoyed when we have someone sick in their machines. You would too if you'd had to do CPR inside a large doughnut.

'He had a fall from a ladder a week ago, with multiple injuries including spinal and rib fractures and an open ankle fracture. Overnight, he was desaturating [meaning his oxygen levels were dropping dangerously low], which they thought may have just been due to his rib fractures but when that didn't get better with painkillers and oxygen, someone thought PE.' When you have major trauma like this, you're quite immobile. And when you're immobile, your blood can clot in places it shouldn't, causing clots in the legs called deep vein thrombosis or economy-class syndrome since they can occur while you're immobile on long-haul flights. These clots can then fly off and cause clots in the lungs, called pulmonary embolus or PE.

The ICU doctor continued. 'He's very unstable. His blood pressure is low and sats are low' (referring to his low oxygen levels again). A PE obstructs blood to your lungs, which can place enormous strain on the heart and take a whole chunk of lung offline, making it hard to take in oxygen. 'Now, I just wanted to know what your thoughts are on embolectomy for this kind of situation?'

My thoughts? 'For it. I'm on my way,' as I sprinted back up my street and straight into my garage. As my car started, I rang my registrar and told him to get into the hospital and get the whole team in, because we were going to be oper- ating in the very near future. I parked my car right outside ED, and felt lucky to be wearing running gear as I sprinted into the hospital and into the CT scanner, where the man was looking decidedly unwell.

I looked at him, I looked at his scans and made a decision in just a few minutes. He needed surgery now. 'All right,' I announced to the room, 'let's get him out of here and up to theatre.' I held his hand and told him that everything would be fine. Which took me by surprise. I never tell patients that everything will be fine. I only ever say that we'll do our very best and take the very best care of them, because I have absolutely no way of knowing that everything is going to be fine.

The trolley bundled from ED to theatre with an inordinate number of people surrounding him. If you want to make someone look sick, I'd recommend wheeling them through the hospital with half a dozen staff members looking concerned and harried. As the theatre door swung open, I was relieved to see the team already there, opening instruments and drawing up drugs out of little glass vials. Each and every person was busy as we got the man off the trolley and onto the table in theatre. It wasn't hectic or uncontrolled; it was organised chaos, everyone moving with pace and purpose.

As the patient was about to go to sleep, I told my registrar that we need to be scrubbed and ready to go in case that process destabilised him. Medications used for anaesthesia, while very safe, can drop your blood pressure. And if your blood pressure is already low, it can cause it to bottom out and, in extreme cases, even trigger a cardiac arrest.

In extreme cases, like that man. It turned out I might have jinxed us all by promising that everything would be fine, because suddenly the arterial line measuring blood pressure took a downward turn and the ECG monitoring of his heart showed the heart slowing to a dangerous level. As I finished throwing on my gown and gloves one of the nurses was already on his chest, jumping up and down trying to deliver blood to his vital organs with CPR. The anaesthetists were giving lifesaving drugs. And the scrub nurse, my registrar and I were splashing antiseptic on his chest and quickly unwrapping drapes.

It took me just a few minutes to get into his chest. It's a strange moment during an emergency. I can hear everything around me, my senses on guard for any signs of trouble. I'm not even sure that I was breathing or just holding my breath the entire time. I took each stitch that my brilliant nurse passed me, ready to secure the pipes to connect him to the heart–lung bypass machine, acutely aware that the blood pressure was still dangerously low. My registrar gently squeezed the heart in between passes of the needles to give a few beats of internal CPR. But it didn't take us long to have his heart connected to the pipes and his circulation safely in the hands of the perfusionist at the heart–lung machine.

'How long?' I called out, wanting to know for how long his brain had potentially been without oxygen while we invaded his chest. The anaesthetist fiddled some buttons on the screen, trying to pinpoint the moments when the blood pressure fell to when the heart–lung bypass machine was in effect. 'I'd say maybe six minutes?' That should be safe for his brain, I thought. 'Pretty fast, maybe faster than the boys!' he told me. I laughed, although honestly right then I didn't care about a pissing contest. There were more important things at hand.

With the heart safely supported, I opened up the left and right pulmonary arteries in turn, squeezing out the biggest clots obstructing both lungs. The clots lay out in a beautiful yet deadly tree, making a perfect cast of the inside of his lungs' most important blood vessels. As I looked at them all, I couldn't help but remark how lucky he was to be alive.

When the patient was safely back in ICU, I went to find his wife, whose face was blotchy and red from crying in the relatives' waiting room. I told her the good news: that her husband had made it safely through surgery and, if all went well, the ICU would be able to wake him up tomorrow morning or even that night. She hugged her child close and said through happy tears, 'Daddy is going to be okay,' before turning and hugging me. I felt tears well up in my eyes so I excused myself and left them to hug each other with enormous relief that it was nothing but good news.

As I walked back to my office, I knew that this was why we put up with all the shit. Why I had worked like a dog that week, and every other week for that matter. It was always for the patients. But I couldn't shake another feeling, that eventually even that gratitude from families could stop being enough to cancel out all of the bad things that happen. Or, more importantly, that we shouldn't be relying on the career highs like that to offset the all-pervading lows and stressors that seemed to become more frequent with each passing year.

I sat down at my computer to compose an email to everyone involved that morning.

Dear all,

I just wanted to write to say thank you for your
excellent work this morning on the gentleman with the
PE. Without everyone's diligence from start to finish, we
may not have had such a good outcome. It's a pleasure
to work with you all; cases like this just serve as a
reminder of what a strong team we have here.

As I typed it, I wondered why we didn't do this more often
and I was just as guilty as the next person. Hospital life
had broken so many of us that, instead of writing an email
to congratulate, we were more likely to denigrate others
for a job we think should have been done better. I'd seen
many more emails complaining about jobs poorly done; no
wonder we needed to wait for the high of a dramatic lifesaving surgery to feel good about ourselves.

The next day, I was still riding high from our successful
surgery. My emotions were on a constant roller-coaster these
days, at the mercy of whether work was a good day or a bad
day. The good days only ever came from great surgeries like
that; the bad days were inevitably about arguments between
colleagues and trying to being on the receiving end.

My phone rang. The very sound of it made me irration-
ally angry, and I was shocked at how quickly my mood
changed from jovial to pissed off. The week had been so
painfully long that I was in a state of anxiety about what
might come bundling through the door next, leaving me
and my one remaining colleague further stretched. But it

wasn't a call about a dramatic emergency. It was far worse than that.

One of my old colleagues from over east was on the line; we had been registrars together. We had suffered through some of the hardest conditions in the country together: long hours, angry bosses and shitty pay. We kind of had a sur-vivors' club with some of the other registrars from the time, laughing about the bad old days over cheap dinners with even cheaper wine. The dark humour and food distanced us from the pain. There were no dark jokes today, though. He barely even said hello, just opened with, 'Did you hear about . . .'

Our old friend.

I could feel my heart start to race as I gingerly asked, 'No, what about her?' I think I knew where it was going, and I knew it wasn't good.

'Oh shit, Stamp. She was found last night.' My brain was struggling to keep up. Found, found where? I thought as the penny dropped. She had died. My colleague continued, 'She's been off work for a while; the head of department knew she wasn't doing so well so they got her some leave to deal with her issues but her brother found her last night at home and . . .' His voice trailed off. I started sobbing, guttural noises so disruptive that everyone in the office came straight to me as I tried to hang up the phone, saying that I was okay, that I'd call back later.

I wasn't okay, as I tried to explain between gasps what had happened to the small crowd of my co-workers surrounding me. 'Why didn't I call?' I asked the room. 'I hadn't spoken to her in four months, why didn't I call? I should have called. I should have called.' My registrar had her arm around my shoulders as out of the corner of my eye I saw people walk into the room and then straight back out when they saw what was happening.

'Go home,' my registrar said, 'we'll be fine without you.' I wasn't operating that day but I couldn't risk leaving the only other surgeon there unaided.

'No,' I insisted. 'I need to be here.' I think that I needed to be there out of a sense of duty but also because I knew that if I went home right then I'd spend the day alone and devastated. If I stayed at work, I could find distractions and human interaction that would dull the pain.

I was awake all night that night, just crying silently, tears rolling down my temples as I lay in bed staring at the ceiling. I opened my phone and found the last text messages we'd exchanged.

How you going? Staying out of trouble I hope ha!

That had been four months before. She had rung me rather than replying and she had sounded exactly as she always did on the phone: happy, hopeful, with just the right amount of cheek. I always found myself in fits of laughter during our conversations. Why hadn't I called again in the last four months? Had I really been that busy and important that I couldn't take twenty seconds out of my day to send her a text? I was supposed to be her friend and mentor and now I felt like I had completely failed her.

A week later, I boarded a flight so that I could attend her funeral. I loved going back to Sydney with my old friends and colleagues, but there wasn't an ounce of pleasure to be obtained on this occasion. I just felt empty inside.

At her funeral, I sat among my old co-workers as we tried to buoy each other's spirits with anecdotes about the time she did this or that or what a brilliant doctor she had been. What a loss to her patients past and future. And while that was absolutely true, I had this horrible sense of unease that her main defining feature was as a brilliant doctor, a talented surgeon. Is this all that we were? Listening to this, it certainly seemed that way. As the service got under way, I looked up at her face on the screen. I should have called, I thought to myself over and over again. I should have called and made sure everything was all right.

After the service, we all mingled and tried to offer some form of comfort to each other. As we stood in a huddle, one of our old bosses came up to join the conversation. I was filled with immense discomfort as I was almost immediately transported back to when we had been in theatre together, and she and I had been helping him do a case. He had called her a fucking moron that day. It felt incredibly wrong that he was there offering condolences when his behaviour had certainly tainted her mental health and that of a number of people there.

I wished I'd called her to see if she was all right. I wished that I was all right.

* * *

I first saw a psychologist to deal with work stress. I saw that same psychologist to support me through my marriage ending but I kept going because of work. It was always about work. In fact, I'd bet that if I tallied up the time that I spent talking about work and how to deal with all the problems that it brought, it would have taken up at least 90 per cent of my visits. Probably took up a large chunk of discussions with family and friends too.

The popular understanding is people go to therapy to talk about their messy marriages and complicated childhoods, but not me. I went to therapy predominantly to deal with my job. I saw a meme once that said, 'I go to therapy to deal with the people in my life who refuse to go to therapy,' and thought that was an apt and amusing description of my situation.

On only one occasion did I talk to my therapist about some of the difficult clinical scenarios I had come across. I cannot even remember how it came up but she asked me about dealing with death at work. And as she did, I was shocked as the list of people whom I had seen die came flooding out of me. I was even more shocked at how sad that list made me. She asked me if I had ever cried at work while telling someone the terrible news that they themselves were dying or that their loved one had died.

The answer was never, ever in front of a patient—which struck us both as decidedly detached. 'It's just not what you do; we're always told to be just a little distant and unemotional lest we're seen as unprofessional.'

She looked me in the eye and said, 'Nikki, if it were me, I'd find some comfort in my doctor being emotional. I'd know they care.'

But by far and away what we discussed the most was not the clinical difficulties. It always came down to talking about managing all of the things that weren't about patient care: all the damaging politics and toxic culture of the workplaces I found myself immersed in. It always felt like I was going around in circles; things were wrong but I had no idea how to fix them. Was it perhaps that they couldn't be fixed but I was too stupid to see it so I insisted on fighting an unwinnable battle? It was beginning to feel like, in the process of trying to change things, the only thing happening was that I was getting increasingly cynical and martyring myself.

We talked about my friend who died, as I poured out my anger and grief to the therapist. Anger at a system that fails time and time again to support doctors when they are tired or vulnerable and then blames them when they falter. Instead, we just keep throwing yoga at the problem and telling ourselves to be more resilient. I listed off the problems that we face: interpersonal difficulties, death, the pressure to perform, job insecurity, the financial strain of becoming a specialist, bullying and sexual harassment, and realised that while I was talking about the things that 'we' as a profession face I was really talking about all of the things that had bothered me. My anger was replaced by intense sadness. 'We all get into this because we love it. I could not have survived surgical training without absolutely loving it. And I do.'

My therapist nodded in agreement. 'But what does it say about a system, a job, even a group of people, that can erode such enthusiasm? That's an impressive feat,' I said with an enormous amount of sarcasm.

My therapist looked at me.

'You don't have to do this job forever.'

She may as well have spoken to me in another language. That was just an idea I couldn't understand, a fate I could never foresee. I was here, forever. I couldn't just quit or give up. Who would I be if I wasn't a surgeon? My biggest fear was that if I wasn't a surgeon I would be a nobody. I would be a great, big failure—to myself, to my peers, to my family and friends. I would have wasted over a third of my life if I just upped and left.

'It might be a bigger waste to waste the next two-thirds of your life, though.'

On a Facebook group of doctors, I started to notice lots of posts asking for advice on leaving medicine. More concerningly the overwhelming majority of them cited reasons like bullying or exhaustion; others spoke of how they had been working for many years but were stranded in their career progression. The list of reasons was almost exclusively confined to finally having had enough of working in an environment that sees breaking you as a character-building exercise or a rite of passage.

* * *

When I got back to work after the funeral, my man with the PE was recovering well. It had been a week and a half since his surgery; his recovery had been a little slow as he dealt with the injuries from his accident and the big cut I had made in the middle of his sternum. But he was finally ready to go home and so I went to see him on the ward. He was so excited for his release from 'jail', as he called it (although the food wasn't as good as prison, he'd joked), that he had packed up all his belongings the night before, ready to escape as fast as he could with his broken bones.

'The wife left something for you and for the nurses,' he said as he handed me a card and a box of my favourite chocolates. I thanked him and immediately got back to business, uncomfortable with the lashings of praise, reminding him to take care of his sternum while it healed. 'You don't really want to see me again, now do you?' I joked as we both laughed.

I took the card and chocolates back to my desk, sharing the chocolates with the office and opening the card.

Thank you for saving my life, Dr Stamp, it read and I pinned it to the board with the rest of the thank you cards received from patients. I took a step back and surveyed them: there were dozens hanging from the board on the wall, and as I looked around the room I saw more of the same on everyone's desks. This is why I do this, I thought. Not for the cards, but for these people.

It seemed that thank you cards and gratitude were my yoga, providing a temporary high to conceal what I was ignoring in the hopes that it would go away. At what point would these fixes stop hiding the fact that I was getting increasingly frustrated with the status quo in medicine and increasingly angry at myself for not being able to fix it?

I was too scared to answer that question.

14

END TIMES

Heartless

When I was a registrar, I used to occasionally assist my bosses on weekends or my days off if they had a case at the private hospital. It seemed like the land of milk and honey there; people were generally so pleasant to each other, the wards were never overflowing with patients spilling out into the corridors and I even got lunch on days I was there. I'd been stalking the halls of that private hospital since I was just a tadpole but, nowadays, I was back there as the boss, working between there and the public hospital.

It was the exact same place and the exact same people who had been there since I was just a bright-eyed young doctor. Going there felt like a warm hug, spending time with the team who had been a feature of my professional life since the beginning. Back then, as I had followed my bosses around as they did their rounds and helped with their surgeries, I had one day imagined myself doing the exact same thing, emulating their careers, their successes and their ability to touch people's lives, some days even save them. And now I was the boss.

As I walked through the doors of this familiar hospital I grinned from ear to ear, feeling like this was exactly where I wanted to be.

Except that behind the smile, things were not going well. What had once been my dream job had now become more akin to something to be endured. It felt like every day I was battling just to stay afloat. Everywhere I looked, I saw so many problems at work. The constant bickering and fighting between colleagues, the sexism that coloured virtually every-thing we did, the broken healthcare system. I saw so many wrongs and I had no idea how to fix them.

Some time at the private hospital, a change of scenery from the public teaching hospital, seemed like exactly what I needed. Any chance I got to operate at the private hospital made me happy, an increasingly challenging thing to do at that point.

I had been referred a man who had dreadfully tight block-ages in his coronary arteries, giving him angina that had been getting worse for weeks on end. His wife had finally convinced him that he needed to go to hospital, after he had dismissed her pleas for too long on the what he hoped never to hear—it *was* something serious.

His ECG, the electrical tracing of the heart, showed that he had suffered a heart attack at some point in the past, maybe in the last few weeks when he had been having pain.

Instead of a quick visit to the ED to appease his wife, he was about to have a pretty serious hospital stay. A battery of tests on his heart showed that he had extremely bad disease in his coronary arteries and that it would be much safer if he had surgery before he went home. He was transferred to the private hospital at his request, which I appreciated for the extra work. Moving patients to the private hospital also had the added bonus of helping to ease the load in the perpetually overworked public hospital. Over half of surgeries in Australia are performed in private hospitals—without them, the public hospital system would buckle further.

When I went to see him on the ward of the private hospital where he had been transferred for surgery, he was so thrilled to see me. Not me, specifically, but after resisting seeing a doctor for his chest pain for so long, he now just wanted to get it sorted and go home. The nurse in his room and I were amused that someone was so thrilled to have heart surgery. Not everyone has that reaction; most would prefer to run the other way and never see us again, in the nicest possible way.

Despite his cheery and robust-looking exterior (he had been a farmer most of his life), as we spoke we uncovered a whole host of issues that were taking his surgery from relatively routine to potentially complicated. Turned out his chest pain wasn't the only thing that he had been ignoring. His wife, sitting next to him on the other side of the hospital bed, looked over her glasses and shook her head at him. I was sure that her frustration with him hid a significant amount of concern.

In the thirty minutes we spent chatting, examining his body and reviewing his tests and notes, some serious problems were discovered. It turned out he had been ignoring some symptoms of what was probably diabetes and of peripheral vascular disease, where the arteries of the arms and legs are blocked as well. I also suspected that he might have had a mini-stroke in the past. None of which was good news. It not only meant that he had come to hospital thinking he was fit and well but would be leaving with a whole host of diagnoses, but it also complicated surgery. His risk for developing issues during his surgery had gone up quite a bit and my job had just got exponentially more complicated.

I had to turn him upside down checking for all of these problems, ordering an enormous battery of tests so that I could not only plan my surgery but also be able to tell this salt-of-the-earth gentleman what he was getting himself in for.

But as the results of all of these tests rolled in, it felt more about what *I* was getting myself in for. I started to doubt myself. Here was a man, a lovely man with a wife who loved him very much, who was going to throw pretty much every curve-ball imaginable at me. And I began to doubt whether or not I could do it.

I had never really felt this way before. I never got anxious before a surgery, especially not since I had become a consultant. I was always mindful of the gravity of what I was about to do, but never anxious. The only time I had felt true, unbridled anxiety, with my heart racing and hands shaking, was back when I was a registrar and I was harvesting the internal mammary artery for a boss who had once called me a fucking useless moron and the thought of being called that again had been scaring me.

On the day of his surgery, I arrived at the private hospital nice and early, wanting to make sure that not only I saw him before he went to sleep but also to demonstrate to the team that I was reliable and capable. I was intent on avoiding developing the same reputations as my colleagues: always running late, perpetually arrogant. But despite being prepared and professional, I could not shake the anxiety.

As I changed into scrubs my hands shook as I tied the string in my scrub pants, which made me even more anxious. Hands shaking while tying knots did not bode for a surgery that involved tying many more knots in hair-fine sutures on the heart. Once I was dressed, I retreated to the 'consultant only' area of the theatre tearoom, a quiet little nook, and tried to compose myself.

Why was I so anxious? What was happening to me? Should I cancel the surgery?

I rang a friend. I needed to hear someone tell me it was going to be okay. I needed to hear someone tell me to get my shit together.

'Why am I freaking out? I never freak out!' I told her down the phone.

'This guy is a bit complicated, maybe you're stressed about that?' she offered in return, which was absolutely correct. I needed to do a really great job today, be on my A game. But this case was no more complicated than other cases I had done in the past. I had the skills; I had done cases like this and they had gone absolutely fine.

What she said next really hit to the very core of the problem.

'You're scared because you have a complex case in a patient that you really like in an environment where everyone is going to talk shit about you if anything goes wrong.'

Bingo. The constant angst that the political and vexatious nature of my workplace brought me had turned me into a wreck. Hearing that plainly explained strengthened my resolve; I was not about to let petty politics and broken systems affect me and my patient. I was going to pull myself together and do the best possible job I could that day.

I saw this man for his follow-up appointment six weeks after we waved him off from the hospital. He looked amazing, everything was healing well and he was walking four kilometres a day when before a walk to the bathroom would have taken all the energy he had. I checked his wounds and his medication and then said what I always say to my patients: 'You have done so well, so, happily, you never have to see me again, in the nicest possible way!' This surgical dad joke usually elicits a chuckle or very strong agreement, because nobody really ever wants to see a heart surgeon. But today this man had something to say that hit me very hard in my current state of angst.

He took both my hands and looked at me with such earnestness and said, 'Thank you. I knew you were the right surgeon for me because I could tell from the very first moment I met you that you absolutely love what you do and care so much about your patients. We knew that I was in good hands.' And with that he left, and I scurried to close the door to the consult room after him to have a moment to collect myself. He couldn't have possibly known how much I needed to hear someone say that.

I used my elation and gratitude for his kind words to try to push down this little voice that was getting more frequent and much louder.

It was saying, what the hell was wrong with me?

* * *

My phone had run hot all night. This was how a transplant happened, with an infinite amount of organisation needed. Trying to arrange recipients, transport, surgeons, theatres and much more for multiple organs meant that, in the lead-up to the actual retrieval, there were endless phone calls and those phone calls happened almost exclusively overnight. Between the hours of midnight and 4 a.m. I had had no less than five phone calls. Although I was exhausted, I wasn't upset. It was just the nature of the beast and it had to be done.

It was just before seven the next morning and I was yawning in the back of a taxi on my way to another hospital to do the organ retrieval; the heart was coming back to our hospital and the lungs were going interstate for a young woman listed for an urgent transplant. When someone is listed as 'urgent', it means that they're incredibly sick and any suitable organ around the country gets offered to them, going all out to save their life. How could it possibly be a bad day, being involved in something like this?

Once we arrived in the hospital, we rolled through the corridors, carrying two conspicuously large blue eskies which loudly announced to anyone in the know what we were here to do. As the lift doors opened, my phone rang; the donor coordinator wanted to know where I was. 'Just getting into the lift,' I told her. 'I'll literally be a few minutes,' wondering why she was calling me when we were actually a little earlier than our agreed-upon arrival time.

'You need to hurry; the donor is unstable and we don't know why.'

Shit, I thought. If a donor became unstable, meaning their blood pressure was plummeting or their heart was struggling, that could damage the organs, rendering them unusable. And given that the life of at least one of today's recipients was literally hanging in the balance, we couldn't afford this. I smashed the lift button to our level, shouting at it to hurry up as if it could hear the urgency in my voice and get us there sooner. When the doors finally crept open, I raced out of the lift, telling my team to follow me with the equipment while I ran ahead to see what was going on.

The entrance to this hospital's theatre is like Fort Knox, understandably, but it was the last thing I needed right now. I knocked on the window, asking the nurse to let me in, please; I was here for the transplant. 'You're going to have to get changed into our scrubs, not the other hospital scrubs.'

'The donor is unstable,' I explained, 'it is *literally* an emergency!'

'I'll let you in this time, but there won't be a next time, will there?' I sighed in frustration and slipped past her to the theatre where the retrieval was happening, thanking her for letting us in. I immediately regretted showing any signs of frustration, because if she had heard that I'd no doubt get in all sorts of trouble.

I could spot ground zero a mile away: people rushing in and out of the theatre doors, looking serious and concerned. The door swung open and I told the very large team that I'd scrub immediately, as quickly as I could, so I could see what was happening. We can't lose the organs, I thought over and over again. As I washed my hands at the sink, the donor coordinator filled me in on what had been happening. The anaesthetists were struggling to maintain the blood pressure, despite throwing everything they could at the donor. Brain death can do this; when our brains die, our organs will carry on working for a period of time but, eventually, they are flooded with chemical messengers from the damaged brain that inevitably stop them working, even with the best that medicine has to offer.

At the chest I joined the abdominal team who were equally as concerned. As I opened the pericardium with my registrar opposite me, I could feel the room was a-flurry. Phone calls were being made, trying to make plan Bs for the organs and the patients who were supposed to receive them. The anaesthetists were working incredibly hard, battling the dwindling blood pressure. As the pericardium peeled back, the answer revealed itself. The heart was empty, a combination of bleeding from surgery, a clotting system that wasn't working and a brain that couldn't tell the body to hold on to fluid to keep it alive anymore. It wasn't irretrievable, I thought; we could still save these organs. And with the problem identified and the extraordinary work of the entire team, we did. Each and every organ was saved and able to be used, to the enormous credit of every single person who pulled together and worked their magic for that donor and the recipients down the track.

To make sure we got back to our hospital in time, we went in a police car, lights and sirens blaring. I usually loved these rides; the adrenaline rush of racing down streets was my version of an extreme sport. By the time we had finished operating, peak-hour traffic was building and we tried to duck and weave between the morning's commuters, many of whom were surprised by the wailing siren behind them, unable to get out of the way. I was filled with anxiety as we ducked in and out of the traffic, the fingers of one hand digging into the seat and of the other death gripping my seatbelt. Which is not normally how I feel; I've slept in the back of police cars on rides like this. I've even sat in the back grinning like a kid on a carnival ride as the car screams through the city streets.

Why was I feeling so anxious again? I hadn't been anxious when I ran into that theatre to save those organs but, as I got out of the police car, I could feel my heart racing and my legs shaking. It dawned on me that I was anxious because I had needed to almost barge my way into theatre, past the red tape of minutiae about scrubs policies when seven lives needing seven organs had hung in the balance. I was anxious that when I got back to my computer there would be an email asking me to explain why I thought I was so special that I could break protocol.

I didn't think I was special, though I had thought the donor and recipients were.

I tried to push that thought out of my head, because the day still had to go on. As the lift rode up, I tried to concentrate on the next tasks at hand: getting the heart safely to theatre and doing the rest of my operations for the day.

Once the heart was safely in theatre next door and the lungs were tucked onto a flight to save a young person's life, I tried to collect my thoughts before my next case started. It was a nice straightforward coronary artery bypass grafting on a lady I'd met in clinic a few months back. She had been booked for surgery three times. Three times she had been cancelled. Once it was a lack of ICU beds; the next the theatre management had told us that they needed our nursing staff elsewhere due to the chronic nursing workforce shortages. The next time, when it was supposed to be 'third time lucky', a heart transplant took priority.

When I was a registrar at a different hospital, patients were cancelled for reasons like this so often we'd joke that they'd only get their operation once they had been cancelled five times. All those times of working yourself up for surgery, of making plans for time off work or travel to this hospital and of family members' worry. The constant need to phone patients and tell them, often as late as the evening before, that despite the preparation they had gone through for the illness that could threaten their life they'd have to wait a bit longer. Some were angry; some were understanding. One woman I had to cancel on the morning of her surgery, because we had to do a lung transplant, was confused as to why she was getting a lung transplant when her lungs were fine. She just couldn't fathom that she had come into hospital and gotten changed into the standard-issue hospital gown and that someone would tell her, sorry, love. Not today.

After years and years in the public hospital system, where this kind of thing happens all the time, it was starting to get to me. Even though as a consultant I wasn't usually the person delivering this bad news (that was done by our nurses or our registrars), I felt enormous guilt at having to do this while being fully aware of the gravity of having to do so. More than that guilt, I was perpetually fuming at the way that cancelling patients for major lifesaving surgery was just seen as inevitable when more often than not it arose from decisions made by an ever-expanding and increasingly frustrating middle management or chronic shortages of beds or hospital staff members.

Those in power (the middle management) who made the decisions to cancel my patients were never the ones having to explain to a crying woman who lives alone why she would have to wait an indeterminate amount of time for her surgery. Again. Instead, someone in management who had never met my patients would send passive-aggressive emails 'suggesting' that you alter the urgency category of that patient because they would never get their surgery within the prescribed time frame, and when they breached that time it would make our numbers look bad. Because that's what we're here for: to make our numbers look good, not look after people. I'd clearly been mistaken for many years in thinking otherwise.

I would conservatively estimate that at least on half of my operating days I'd spend time negotiating or begging to make sure that all of my cases went ahead. That there would be ICU beds, or anaesthetic technicians or that the theatre maintenance could be done another day that wouldn't cause patients to be cancelled. These pleas so frequently ended with middle management throwing up obstruction after obstruction, letting the hours pass by until it got to be so late in the day it was not as safe as we would want it to be to start major surgery. You'd then have to rebook the case for another day and let the poor patient finally eat something. Management would then record in their computer system that the case was 'cancelled by the surgeon' so that they were absolved of responsibility and it looked like one of the surgeons just couldn't be bothered. After yet another day of fighting to get a case done, to be met with endless hindrances, I shared my frustrations with a theatre coordinator by telling her that if she bowed to bureaucracy and cancelled my afternoon case, she could be the one to go and tell the patient waiting in her hospital gown that she had been cancelled because I was sick of doing it.

I got a complaint for that.

In all honesty, I was probably terse. And I understand that most of us are doing what we can with what we have, but sometimes that isn't much amid the constraints of policies and practices that are not conducive to providing good care.

And yet, any complaint we made about a system that was bursting at the seams was shrugged off as 'just one of those things'. It's impossible to do heart surgery when bureaucracy ties both hands behind your back.

The lady my registrars were helping me with that day had joked as she had gone off to sleep, 'I won't believe I'm actually getting heart surgery until I wake up with a cut in my chest.' The theatre staff laughed and reassured her but, honestly, she had a point. Today was her day though and my two registrars were doing a great job, starting the case while I watched over their shoulders. One was taking the internal mammary artery, the other the radial artery from the left wrist. It was their chance to fly almost solo, with me in the proverbial backseat, pointing out how they could improve this or how the way they used the instruments was perfect. Once they had completed this first part of the operation, I'd take over and do the rest.

I was thankful for the short break, to be able to sit back and observe and teach rather than have to do this part of the surgery myself. The anxiety had abated but the exhaustion hadn't, neither the physical exhaustion from multiple overnight phone calls nor the emotional exhaustion from everything else that was draining my very being.

Surgery was starting to feel like an abusive relationship. I needed the ups or the good times—the heartwarming feeling from saving a life, the thrill of knowing a transplant would grab someone back from the brink of death. I had to have these fixes to try to disguise all the times when it was, little by little, breaking my spirit.

I decided that since this lady needed a relatively straightforward operation, I'd let my registrar finish it. I was so proud of him. He had been my registrar for two years; he had been excellent to start with and was becoming even more outstanding. I took my place on the patient's left side, just like my bosses had done with me years before, and guided him through the surgery. As the last sutures went in, this woman given the bypass grafts she so desperately needed, I could feel tears welling up like a proud parent.

I told him he had done an amazing job, and in return he gave me another fix to dull the pain from the abusive side of my surgical relationship.

'You're an awesome teacher, Nikki; thank you for everything you do for me.'

The heart transplant in the theatre next door had gone smoothly and my afternoon was just a straightforward lung cancer operation. Given that I was tired and, although I'd never admit it (perhaps I hadn't even realised it), I was burnt out to within an inch of my life, a nice relaxing afternoon case was exactly what I needed. Lung surgery was not necessarily easier but it was usually shorter, and when we got to operate on people with lung cancer it gave them a chance to recover from what is a really dreadful disease.

An hour into my nice, quiet afternoon case, as I was consumed by what I was doing, one of my colleagues burst into my theatre. I could tell he was spoiling for a fight, which I needed like a hole in the head. As he entered the room, he strode over to my anaesthetist to argue about why his case had gotten cancelled this afternoon (for a transplant) and how he was fucking sick and tired of being treated so poorly. The yelling was a distraction from what I was trying to do, so without looking up I said, 'Mate, can you please take this outside? I'm operating.'

That was when the shit really hit the fan. A young nurse on her first day in our theatre, scrubbed next to me, stood back from the table, aghast at the expletive-laden rant that had already ensued and seemingly preparing herself for what came next. (She was so horrified that she requested never to come back to cardiac theatre again.)

'Don't you fucking dare talk to me like that. I am a consultant here too and you are fucking rude and will show me some respect . . .' he said to me. And it went on and on like that. He was still standing next to the anaesthetist but his booming voice filled the entire space. His tirade happened while my hand was deep inside someone's chest—deeply unprofessional and unsafe for that patient. I couldn't even retreat from the noise, trapped by my responsibility to my patient and the sterile drapes and gowns.

I did what I thought was best when people throw tantrums, which was to say absolutely nothing until his outburst fizzled out, I assume because he'd called me fucking rude or fucking useless or whatever else enough times to ensure that I got the message. I finished the case through tears welling up in my eyes. I realised that there was a line and this consultant's behaviour had stomped all over it.

After the case was finished I rang my boss, the person whose job it was to do the right thing in that situation—to stand up for me, my patient and what was right. But clearly my colleague had got his call in first. When I got on the phone to the boss and told him what had happened, his response was, 'Look, he's a nice guy. Maybe you need to think about what you did to provoke that behaviour?'

What the hell?

What had I done? I had been looking after my patient, mate. I had silently watched as everyone in the room sat there and did nothing while my so-called peer, my teammate, had decided that the middle of an operation was a good time to come in and swear at me. There was so much that was very, very wrong with this situation. Not least of which was the absolutely disgusting behaviour my colleague thought to unleash on me mid-operation and the woeful inaction from the bystanders. And my boss offering zero support. But what it finally got through to me was that this place was broken, the culture was in the toilet, it lacked leadership and, most importantly, I felt like I wasn't wanted there. I wasn't supported, I wasn't believed and I wasn't valued. And just like that, my heart broke into a million pieces. My dream job was increasingly feeling like a nightmare that I was being forced to repeat every single day.

I tracked down a friend for a debrief, still in disbelief. Over a very late lunch, I told her what had happened. By this stage, I had graduated from tearful heartbreak to outright fury.

'All I want is to do my job. I don't want to have to deal with constant bullshit; why is that so fucking hard?' I lamented. 'Operating is easy. If I could hide away in theatre all day and just operate, I'd be happy. If I could chat to my patients, I'd be happy. But instead, it's fighting for beds or listening to my colleagues behave like five year olds or sexist bullshit or useless rules that do nothing for the actual patients. It's always fucking something.'

I put my head in my hands and tried not to cry from sheer frustration into my overpriced soggy sandwich. On that day, I started to seriously wonder if it was all worth it.

* * *

I was finally home that evening, trying to digest the events of the day. I'd been so distracted by everything that I only now remembered that the lungs I had retrieved that morning were probably by now helping a young woman to breathe again. Or that the heart recipient was now disconnected from a machine keeping him alive, also with the promise of a full life ahead. I had forgotten that my poor lady from this morning who had been cancelled repeatedly had finally gotten her surgery, or that lung cancer patient from the afternoon now had the chance to live cancer free. I was overcome by guilt for getting so wrapped up in my own issues at work when what I really should have been thinking about was the patients.

My self-reproach was interrupted by a text message from one of my former RMOs. She was brilliant, unflappable, intelligent and ambitious and on her way to being a surgeon. We'd had so many chats about her career; she was currently a registrar in another specialty and hadn't been having the greatest time. The overseas fellow treated her like his personal slave, overworking her and throwing her under the bus for any mistake he made. Which meant that consultants looked at her with pity, not promise, which in my opinion was a grave error. For six months, she had put her head down and just gotten on with the job as best as she could in what could only be described as a hostile environment. And for six months I had told her just to hang on, things would get better, she was going to make a wonderful surgeon and that I believed in her.

The message read: *Thanks for all your support but I've decided that I don't want to do surgery anymore.*

My first thought was that I had failed her. I hadn't provided enough support or the right kind of support to help her manage all the stress that was being thrown at her. I hadn't given her the right tools to fight back against the sexual harassment or the bullying from her fellow. I hadn't called her boss and begged him to look out for her because she's painfully talented. I hadn't managed to change the system so that we didn't keep losing brilliant, talented doctors like her.

And then I was filled with intense anger. Anger that surgery had lost such an asset who would now no doubt be dismissed as 'just not suited to surgery' when in truth what she really wasn't suited to was being overworked, underappreciated and treated with such intense disrespect and disdain. She wasn't suited to being at the behest of a system that was dysfunctional and frustrating to the point where it impedes your ability to actually care for patients.

Every time this happens, every time we lose brilliant people like her, I want to tear the system down. I want to dismantle every unjust piece and hold the individuals who perpetuate it accountable. For every leap forward we had made in surgery, it still felt like we took a dozen steps backwards. How could I, in good faith, encourage someone to just keep going when each attempt at toughing out whatever unnecessary obstacle was thrown at you was only met with more obstacles? It would be like convincing someone to stay in an abusive relationship because that was exactly how this was beginning to feel. Along with my anger at a broken system was a part of me that wanted to tell her to run and take her talents somewhere else, somewhere that deserved them.

All of which made me reflect on my own situation. That day had been awful; there is no denying that. But those awful moments and awful days were starting to get more common and I was feeling less equipped to deal with them. The job that I loved so much was now breaking my heart and my spirit. And I started to wonder just how long I could endure it—the bullying, the bureaucracy, the stress, the unfairness, the misery—before it finally broke me. I was tired of fighting, whether it was fighting the system to be able to get the work done, for equality for us and for our patients, or to hold on to a dream I had had as a small girl.

Reflecting back on my career to that point, I realised I hadn't ever really assessed what I had sacrificed, willingly or unwillingly. Totalling up the ledger at that point was a painful assessment for me. Sure, I had gritted my teeth and made it through training in a field that I loved. But at what cost? A marriage (at least in part), relationships, friendships, mental health, significant financial costs, my physical health, having a family, conflict, dealing with death, many hours of sleep and study and intense emotional and sometimes physical isolation.

And now I was thinking, for what? What was it all for? Did I love my job enough to justify these sacrifices, or perhaps more accurately did I love my job enough to continue? The truth is, at this point I didn't know anymore. I had been so strong and tenacious for so long and now I felt like I had unravelled. I just didn't have any more fight left in me.

The tears started to flow freely as the realisation dawned that, while saving other people, I had been dying by a thousand cuts. Every bit of training, every sacrifice, was there for that moment when you could save someone's life.

And now I was almost inconsolable. 'I *was* a really good surgeon,' I sobbed to my partner at the time, feeling like everything I had ever worked for was just gone.

'Nikki, you are a good surgeon. No, a great surgeon. And you love what you do and you love your patients.'

I don't think I can do this anymore.

15

LIVING IN THE MOMENT
The heart will go on

I left my public hospital job in what can only be described as unpleasant circumstances. As I did, I genuinely thought that my world was crumbling. Not only was I losing the thing that got me up in the morning—my patients, the people I saw every day—I was suddenly facing all of the angst that came with leaving a job. The financial stress and the complete lack of security were only compounded by the shame I felt from losing what I thought was the defining part of my identity.

I didn't leave being a surgeon, or my love of the heart or even the patients; I was leaving a toxic workplace. With each year that passed, I was increasingly frustrated by the numerous wrongs I saw in my workplace, day in and day out. As I began to realise just how broken surgery was, I couldn't contain my frustrations any longer. The impossible had been achieved—my love of surgery had been nearly erased.

Although I had attempted to sit down with the hospital to tell them that it was not just a case of a few bad apples but an entirely rotting tree, the only response was that I should have raised it sooner (which would have risked my career) or that my experiences were 'misconceived'.

If I was being honest, none of these things were new. In fact, the problems I saw had been around since the dawn of time, long before I entered the profession. They had certainly been present since I first became a doctor. As a junior doctor, I think I chose to ignore or justify so many of the bad behaviours of people and the brokenness of the system we worked in out of self-preservation, by saying that, on balance, we contributed more to society than we took away from each other. I didn't really think I could change things, but I am heartbroken that I couldn't even make a dent.

If I couldn't survive and I couldn't fix it, how could I stay?

Female doctors leave their profession at alarming rates. Throughout surgical training, women are far more likely to leave surgery, at least twice as likely as their male counterparts, as reported in Australian research published in *The Lancet*. According to US research, after completing their specialist training nearly 40 per cent of women scale back their practice or leave medicine altogether. And they do this not because they dislike being a surgeon. They do it because they are bullied and harassed; they're treated as inferior to their male counterparts, and they are forced to juggle far more, and all of this while doing a job that is demanding in a way that very few other professions can be. And the biggest loss in all this is for our patients. Research published in prestigious medical journals, including the *Journal of the American Medical Association*, shows that female doctors and surgeons are of particular importance to female patients. When they are treated by a female doctor, they have better outcomes from a hospital stay. Female doctors likely pick up on things like social cues or the experience of a woman that might otherwise be lost.

When huge numbers of people are walking away from something they have dedicated at least half their life to that is a huge red flag that there is something very, very wrong with that profession.

For me, life changed dramatically. My days went from being filled with operating and seeing patients to trying (and failing) to establish a private practice where I could continue to do what I loved. I tried to focus on my research, but without a public hospital appointment my entire PhD needed to be rethought, almost starting from scratch.

This meant that I had a lot of free time on my hands to think things through. With that came a roller-coaster of emotions. For most of my life, I had defined myself as a surgeon. When I had to describe myself to someone, I would inevitably describe myself as a surgeon straight off the bat. Away from the operating theatre I felt decidedly adrift, not just in my professional capacity but in my very being. If I wasn't a surgeon then who was I? Which led to a much more frightening question: if I wasn't a surgeon, was I good enough?

While it sounds like a nice break, it hadn't been a planned one. After leaving my last job I did short-term jobs, filling in for colleagues taking holidays and doing a few cases here and there in private hospitals. I thought it would only be a short-term arrangement, but as fate would have it, it went longer than I had initially planned.

Instead of waking up to days defined by the operations I was doing, I was suddenly filling my days with policy and procedure, research and writing. No longer was I stalking the hallways of a hospital at all hours, glued to my phone in case of some emergency or urgent clinical question. And at first I was absolutely lost, cut adrift from the one thing I thought I truly loved and that truly completed me. Despite being as busy as ever, the absence of surgery had left an enormous hole.

At that time, I didn't want to stop being a surgeon; in fact, my days and nights were consumed with plans to move across the country or around the world, to get back to that right-hand side of the patient, surrounded by beeping machines and tubes filled with blood, ready to restore hope where there was none. But, slowly, something began to change as I started to, for the first time ever, really, brutally assess where my life was headed.

Something finally dawned on me while I stopped and took a breath. Maybe I hadn't been as happy as I had thought I had been. As each year had passed, I could now see with hindsight that while I would probably never stop loving the magic of the heart or meeting patients, I had started to dislike my job a little more with each passing year.

None of this despondence was because of the surgery itself. Operating and taking care of people doesn't scare me; I am fully aware of what a wonderful privilege it is to be trusted like that. I was petrified to go back to surgery because of all the other things that we force each other to endure. Nearly two decades of nasty office politics, broken health-care systems, sleepless nights, sexism and feeling powerless to change any of it had taken the sheen off my once beloved career. I am resilient and tough, but in the decades I had spent saving other people it now started to dawn on me that I might have been sacrificing myself slowly in the process.

Voicing this fear and the possibility that I might never go back, not only to cardiac surgery but medicine at all, was just as frightening. It is not the done thing to say that you're so unhappy, you're thinking of leaving. It's quite okay to bemoan the shitty situation you're in but then you just carry on.

I plucked up the courage to ask a friend and colleague for help and advice. In tears down the phone, I told him that I wasn't sure I could do this anymore. A year had passed since I had left my last job and I was doing the bare minimum of cardiac surgery but still couldn't quite find another job or a stable private practice, nor could I reconcile myself to going back into the shark-infested waters of hospital surgical departments.

I heard him sigh down the phone.

'I understand why you'd feel that way but honestly, that is a fucking travesty. You have been squeezed from every side in recent years and it's a huge loss.'

Yes, it was. I saw myself as losing everything I had worked for, not least of all my love of my job and my admiration for those who did it. But I also started to realise that the only greater loss would be if I continued in a job that was making me sick and unhappy. But I remained unconvinced that I could completely walk away.

'We need to stop just pulling people out of the river. We need to go upstream and find out why they're falling in.'

—Archbishop Desmond Tutu

Medicine, and surgery in particular, has a blind spot when it comes to looking at its own shortcomings. In 2015, a female Sydney vascular surgeon was overheard by a journalist dryly saying that for a woman in surgery to be successful, she would be better off giving in to any sexual advances from her bosses lest she sacrifice her career. What ensued was a very public airing of the surgery's dirty laundry, with major media outlets in Australia and overseas delving into the dark underbelly of bullying and sexual harassment that had been normalised and gone unchecked.

This public reckoning forced surgery in Australia to undertake a very long, painful and expensive assessment of bullying, discrimination and sexual harassment in the profession. As a result, the Royal Australasian College of Surgeons rolled out new standards and training to try to purge these kinds of behaviours from our profession.

Noble as its efforts have been, the sad fact is that medicine and surgery are so steeped in problems that five short years of effort by one part of the healthcare system are not enough to undo the vast problems that face our profession.

Nobody comes into medicine unaware of the pressures of the job. We are all fully prepared for the inevitable downsides of medicine, like losing patients, making mistakes and working so hard you feel tired deep in your soul. This is not a shock to us and it is something that we can overcome, because for every sad or tragic event there are far more wins. We alleviate suffering far more than we fail at it. We save many more lives than we cannot and we make the right moves infinitely more often than we ever make errors.

What breaks us is far more insidious and difficult to overcome. The years of sexism, much of which I wilfully ignored or summarily dismissed as a junior doctor, grew to be a huge black cloud above my head. Year after year I realised just how medicine, and surgery in particular, mistreat their female doctors through beliefs and practices that are so ingrained they seem natural.

I wish I had spoken up years ago but I believed that I was tough enough to survive in that environment. Other times, I realised that explaining that your boss was making filthy jokes in theatre was signing your own career's death warrant. And worst of all, there were far too many times when I excused that behaviour because I was so captivated by the amazing work these people were doing. Now I am full of guilt, because every time I didn't speak up I left the door open for mistreatment to happen to other people and for these patterns to become even more deeply ingrained.

Hospitals and health systems have long blamed rogue doctors and badly behaved surgeons in these situations because it conveniently shifts blame away from their own shortcomings. Working in a system that is always stretched to breaking point is soul destroying. Year after year, you fight with hospital administrators and ever-growing layers of inept middle management to get your work done. Try to change or improve the system and you're met with incredible resistance, with explanations of how it's too hard, there's no money or the age-old 'we've always done it that way'.

Hospitals know that people who work in health care are good people. You just do not become a doctor, or any kind of healthcare professional for that matter, if you don't care about helping people. Managers and administrators know this and exploit it to the point where you're working for free, too scared to ask for the overtime that kept you at work for several hours after your shift was up. It keeps you from taking a holiday when you haven't had one in years because your department will be left short and you don't want to be the person who shafts your colleagues and your patients.

None of these problems is unique to surgery. Every medical specialty has these problems, some to a greater or lesser degree, but they are there. Neither are the hands of everyone else at the hospital clean. Whether you're a doctor, a nurse or any other healthcare worker, for a group of people who wanted to do the best for someone we are all experiencing the same pressures and we all have a propensity to treat each other badly.

I like to think that we all started out in medicine with truly honourable intentions. What makes me sad is that year after year, all these other pressures in an unforgiving and at times toxic environment tarnish those good intentions. We're taught that enduring bad behaviours—like yelling at people for sport or sexual harassment—are just 'what it takes' to be a surgeon. And while these behaviours break our spirits or allow us to think that this is acceptable, it may even tarnish our fascination and enjoyment for a job that we once loved. I don't want to be like that, and I am afraid that if I stay that would be my fate.

We should all care that we break or lose so many wonderfully talented doctors. I have been a patient, and I have been a relative of patients. I don't want someone looking after me who is disillusioned, resigned, cynical. I want someone who still has a passion and a fire for what they do and is free to do their job without fear, without restriction and without unnecessary pain. When it comes to wanting the best for our doctors, trust me, we all have skin in this game.

***

It was strange at first, not heading to an operating theatre every day. I threw myself into all of my other work—writing, research, advocacy. Although away from the stress of a hospital and the demanding nature of my work in some ways I blossomed, I still found myself wrestling with what I was going to do next with my life. Increasingly, I found myself wanting to leave medicine altogether. Not because I hated it but because I began to think that the only way to change it was from the outside.

As COVID-19 devastated the world, part of me was healed. I started working in general medical jobs, where I met with a variety of medical issues, most of which were small and which I could therefore help with far simpler remedies than open-heart surgery. I was reminded of how good it feels to alleviate someone's symptoms. Exposure to an incredible breadth of issues reminded me just how amazing the human body was. It also reminded me how wonderful medicine can be. Trust me, had it not been for that I had been ready to walk away from medicine altogether.

At the time, as it became clear what I needed to do, a few people were astonished. 'After all this time, what a waste!' even some of those closest to me would exclaim. But the only real waste would be if I stayed in a job that was making me sick, unhappy and, most importantly, unable to change the things about medicine, surgery, hospitals and health care that so desperately needed to be remedied. Within the system I was powerless to a degree, beholden to a culture that simultaneously kept you down and punished you for being different or for speaking up. That would be the real waste of my passion, my talent and my sense of right and wrong.

With the gifts of some distance and time from surgery, I noticed two very important lessons. The first was that nobody could ever erase my love for medicine and surgery completely. I will never stop wanting to save people and make their lives better. The second and very important thing for me to realise was that I was happier than I had ever been. With that came an understanding that I deserved this happiness, but also a sense of clarity about what I wanted to do next in my life. As I write this, I still cannot say for certain what my future holds, except to say that I am not leaving medicine but I am going to change what I do within it.

I wanted to be a doctor to make the world a better place, and being a heart surgeon, I had thought, was the best way for me to do that. Being a heart surgeon is a wonderful job; although the system is broken and the people are imperfect, I don't have regrets. Had I known what I know now, I hope that I would have made different decisions. I am so grateful for the skills and experience I have gained and for the many wonderful people I have met, both colleagues and patients alike. And make no mistake, although this book has chronicled some of the worst moments, even those who are falling short of expectations are still out there every day doing good. And like me, they're doing it in a system and a culture that is in desperate need of radical change on so many fronts.

My experience and my skills will never be wasted. And I will never stop being a doctor nor will I ever stop being fascinated by, and an expert in, the heart. What I am going to do with that knowledge and experience, though, that is the exciting part.

In my more cynical moments, I have felt that the healthcare system is beyond healing. I have also wondered if there are any good people still left in it. I've wondered if it is worth fighting for.

It is—there is so much worth fighting for. And more than ever, I want to do just that.

I want a healthcare system where its workers are valued and nurtured and where we all realise that we are so much better than the sum of our parts. I want health care to be for all people, and to strive every day to do what it actually exists to do—help others. I want for us all to be able to do our jobs without red tape and toxic environments that hamper our ability to care for our patients and ourselves. I want medicine to be as decent as it claims to be, because once upon a time even the most jaded of us wanted to truly help people.

One thing is certain and that is, whatever I end up doing, I know that I still want to save the world. And that is exactly what I'm going to do.

EPILOGUE

January 2022

Over the course of the past two years as I have written this book, I have spent countless hours reflecting deeply on everything I have seen and experienced. During that time it has been hard not to feel deep, aching pain for the lowest of lows that I experienced. And it is equally hard not to deeply yearn that things were different.

How did this happen? How did I get here? Hell, how did we all get here? It's almost unfathomable that a group of people who largely started on this pathway in medicine and surgery could be anything other than kind. After all, we exist every day to make people better. What happens to make people do almost the exact opposite?

I can only come to one answer.

In my profession, we take people who have a passion and we put those people in the most austere environment imaginable. We ask surgeons to take on the heady responsibility of being responsible for another's wellbeing, even their lives. We ask them to do so in a healthcare system that is stretched beyond its capabilities and poisoned by politics. We ask them to sacrifice everything—their own health, family, sleep—and make sure that asking for help or even stumbling is a sign of weakness. All the while, our teachers role model destructive ways of dealing with this pressure—doing unto others as was done unto them. We celebrate bravado and arrogance, because it seems to be the only way to succeed in a system that beats so many of us down at every opportunity.

Surgeons and doctors are not bad people, but we risk being tainted by a system and a culture that is most certainly rotten.

It might seem surprising after the events detailed in the pages of this book to say that the very same people who can reduce you to tears are the same people who have shed tears for a patient and begged and pleaded with God to spare someone's life as they fight gallantly against disease. They're the same people who have been my friends and colleagues, my teachers and mentors and expressed pride in what I and others have achieved. They support charitable causes and give time and expertise to those who need it most.

What reflection has taught me is that nobody is all good or all bad. But I am certain that years of dealing with the very real and unrelenting pressures of being a surgeon in these environments amplify some of the worst parts of any of us.

How do I know this with such certainty? Because I knew that if I stayed, this would be me too. Understanding these complexities has allowed me to look at everything that has happened with compassion and with forgiveness.

As I started writing this book, I found myself at a fork in the road. I could take one pathway and continue on in a career that was devastating me, physically and emotionally, clawing my way back to what I had wanted since I was a child, and that was exactly what I tried to do. But as I tried to do so, the cynicism and hostility in me was no longer bubbling beneath the surface, it was consuming me.

This realisation forced me to examine the other pathway. And, ultimately, I have found my peace on this road.

Even though the path I have chosen has seen me 'leave' surgery, I haven't entirely. I still do some surgery, but instead of it being a source of pain it's like a weight has been lifted. For now I have no plans to return to full-time surgical practice, but I will never stop being a surgeon. I'll never stop being a doctor. In fact, in the moment that I finally decided it was time to leave full-time surgery and move on, I found more peace and happiness than I can ever remember experiencing. Most importantly, I have a renewed sense of purpose and, unlike my desperation to be a heart surgeon, the anxiety about achieving my next goal just isn't there.

So, what is next for me? I have never been someone to sit idly by when I see a problem. Throughout the last twenty-odd years of medical school and medical practice, I have seen so many opportunities for making the healthcare system better for patients and doctors alike, so that is exactly what I'm going to do.

Since I 'left' surgery, I have continued to advocate for health care for women, specifically for women's heart disease. I've continued to do the same for women in medicine, so that we can continue to attract the best and brightest. The biggest change I have made, though, is to move towards a career in medical administration, where instead of being at the behest of the system I may have a chance to make it better. And who knows where that will take me? Maybe all the way to running health care for the whole country one day; only time will tell.

The one thing I can tell you with the greatest certainty is that the past is in the past and I am going to make the future brighter for as many people as I possibly can.

Lastly, and this is the most important thing for me right now, I am absolutely and completely happy. After all this time, I did something I had nearly failed at during my career. I have finally saved myself.

ACKNOWLEDGEMENTS

When I first started writing many years ago, I was not sure if I would ever write a book like this. It seemed self-indulgent—why was my story important when so many people have achieved far greater things than I have? However, when the opportunity to tell this story arose, I started to realise how important it is to tell the story of surgery so that it may be able to heal itself.

This book has taken the better part of two years to write in a process that has been nothing short of difficult—it has been deeply personal, confronting and painful at times. And it would not have happened without the help of many people.

My publisher, Tom Gilliatt, has been instrumental in guiding me to make this book the best that it can be. I'm very grateful for his expertise and patience with me. Tom Bailey-Smith and Susan Keogh did such a remarkable job editing the manuscript to take it to another level. The entire team at Allen & Unwin have been wonderful from the beginning and I thank them for this.

Simone Landes and the rest of the team at The Lifestyle Suite provided much support and championing of this and all the other work I do as always, and I can't thank you all enough.

Although I didn't write this book under her guidance this time, Jane Morrow has been a champion from the sidelines. After two books, Jane, you made me think I might actually be able to do this and I hope this book makes you proud.

To the patients I have come across in my career, whether I met you last week or more than twenty years ago when I was just a medical student, you are my heroes. I wish I had half the courage you all did and I want to thank you for being my reason for getting out of bed every day and my reason for wanting medicine to be the best it can be.

I have had so many wonderful colleagues over the years. Even those who are flawed have taught me so much about medicine and life. For those of you who have been friends, colleagues, teachers, confidants and cheerleaders, thank you.

While I was writing this book, my friends were peppered with questions and gave advice and support in return. I could not be luckier to have such wonderful people in my life.

To the fur babies, Lola and Harry, you give the best snugs, which made writing much easier.

Finally to my family—my parents and Nathan, Nikki, Jesse (and the little one on the way)—you are the very best.